THE PSYCHOLOGY OF ALFRED ADLER AND THE DEVELOPMENT OF THE CHILD

Founded by C. K. Ogden

The International Library of Psychology

INDIVIDUAL DIFFERENCES
In 21 Volumes

THE PSYCHOLOGY OF ALFRED ADLER AND THE DEVELOPMENT OF THE CHILD

MADELAINE GANZ

Introduction by Pierre Bovet

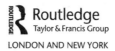

LONDON AND NEW YORK

First published in 1953 by
Routledge and Kegan Paul Ltd

Reprinted 1999, 2000, 2001 by
Routledge
2 Park Square, Milton Park, Abingdon, Oxon, OX14 4RN
Simultaneously published in the USA and Canada by Routledge
711 Third Avenue, New York, NY 10017

Transferred to Digital Printing 2006

Routledge is an imprint of the Taylor & Francis Group, an informa business

First issued in paperback 2013

© 1953 Madelaine Ganz, Translated by Philip Mairet

The publishers have made every effort to contact authors/copyright holders
of the works reprinted in the *International Library of Psychology*.
This has not been possible in every case, however, and we would
welcome correspondence from those individuals/companies
we have been unable to trace.

These reprints are taken from original copies of each book. In many cases
the condition of these originals is not perfect. The publisher has gone to
great lengths to ensure the quality of these reprints, but wishes to point
out that certain characteristics of the original copies will, of necessity, be
apparent in reprints thereof.

British Library Cataloguing in Publication Data
A CIP catalogue record for this book
is available from the British Library

The Psychology of Alfred Adler and the Development of the Child

ISBN 978-0-415-21056-0 (hbk)
ISBN 978-0-415-86887-7 (pbk)

It matters little what we bring into the world, everything depends on what we make of it.

A. ADLER

Contents

vii

CONTENTS

A

Preface

MADEMOISELLE MADELAINE GANZ asks me for a preface to a book which, after being awarded the Lucien Cellérier prize by the University of Geneva, has gained for her the degree of Doctor of Philosophy. I have no qualification for introducing the work beyond having been its instigator and first reader. Having no personal knowledge of the institutions to which she has devoted her study, I will limit myself to saying why I am happy to welcome it into our *Collection d'Actualités Pédagogiques* and to place this monograph beside those which have so far attained that distinction.

Mlle. Ganz's intelligent and attentive description of the Adlerian schools and consultative methods comes as a timely addition to the accounts which Mr. Anderson and Mme. Loosli have given us of the Healy psychological clinic, and of the medico-psychological consultations at the Institut J. J. Rousseau.[1] Far from rendering each other redundant, these monographs will arouse in their readers a desire for information about other social services of the same kind. Why should we not also be told of the procedure at Leipzig and at Paris, at Guy's Hospital in London and at the observational station at Moll? Is it not encouraging to see that this work is proceeding on every hand, and singularly instructive to compare the methods employed? What at first sight chiefly distinguishes psychological-pedagogical consultations from one another is the position

---

[1] H. H. Anderson, *The Psychological Clinics for Children in the United States and the Work of Dr. Healy.* 1929. Marguerite Loosli-Usteri, *Les enfants difficiles et leur milieu familiale. L'activité d'une consultation médico-pedagogique.* 1935.

that they accord respectively to methods of gaining information; interrogation, clinical examination, experimentation or, to name only the two most controversial procedures, tests on the one hand, and, on the other, investigation into the subconscious. We have seen in Healy's work the considerable place assigned to tests of the most varied kinds; Mme. Loosli, who has acquired eminent competence in the application of the Rorschach test to children, has shown us how serviceable she has found this method, of a psychoanalytic tendency, in conjunction with others that seek to measure the aptitudes and the level of intelligence. With Adler, it is the interpretation of behaviour, as a function of desires for the most part unconscious, to which the greatest importance is attached.

May I state, briefly, from my personal experience, the present position in relation to concrete cases of this recourse to the psychology of deeper levels—to what the Germans call 'Depth-psychology'. It was a great satisfaction to me, at the Congress of the New Education held in South Africa in 1934, to see my experience exactly confirmed by the far wider experience of Boyd from Glasgow.

People send us children whose school records are wholly deplorable: their orthography, arithmetic, their German or Latin, or what you will—are so poor that we are asked whether some exercises in concentration, some kind of orthophrenic gymnastics are not indicated. We begin by simply measuring the intellectual capacity of the child according to the classic scale of Binet (and I do not yet understand how informed practitioners, those of Vienna for example, can voluntarily deprive themselves of such information as this affords). Frequently we find that the child's mental level is perfectly normal, that its intelligence quotient exceeds 100: one cannot ascribe its want of success at school to mental backwardness. The intelligence is not in question. Can it be, then, an emotional disequilibrium that is troubling the child's attention to study? The Rorschach test is of service in distinguishing any such instability. Other instruments of research are employed elsewhere. Boyd makes use, with great success, of a list of associations inspired by Jung. We can also tell whether it will be prudent to confide the further interrogation of the child to a psychiatrist, or whether the instability thus betrayed is such as an examination of the child's family and social surroundings can clarify, by placing ourselves at one or another of the points of view recommended by the diverse schools of psychoanalysis.[1]

Of these standpoints, as M. Claparède has lately demonstrated,[2] that of Adler is one of the most useful. And this monograph by Mlle. Ganz, which provides such an intelligent selection of such varied examples, will certainly be of great assistance to the practical psychologist and educator.

It goes without saying that general medicine has, in any case, its own contribution to make.[3] There is no further need to plead in favour of the medical examination of the difficult child. In every case one will also inquire into its material circumstances. Of this the recent book by Mme. Kaczinska[4] has once again shown the immense importance.

We are here concerned with schoolchildren, but our scholastic buildings have not, unfortunately, any monopoly in 'difficult children'. The phrase is nearly related to another—the 'problem child', which in Anglo-Saxon countries is by way of becoming a technical term. But so to describe the 'difficult children' of the family and the school becomes, after their school-leaving age, a euphemistic term

[1] Ch. Baudouin, *L'ame enfantine et la psychanalyse.* 1931.
[2] Ed. Claparède, *Le sentiment d'infériorité chez l'enfant* (*Cahiers de pédagogie expérimentale No. 1*). Geneva. 1934.
[3] See the interesting preface by Claparède to the book by Mme. Loosli mentioned above.
[4] M. Kaczinska, *Succès scolaire et l'intelligence.* 1934.

for those young delinquents whom the Belgians call 'children of justice'. The problems grow more difficult, the social disadaptation more flagrant, but the factors of misbehaviour remain the same, and therefore a psychological diagnosis of the case is also still necessary. This is not yet everywhere understood. It is but a few weeks since, at Geneva, a new regulation was imposed upon the Penal Court for Children, in which it was not possible to obtain the incorporation of the principle of obligatory medico-psychological examination. This must come, however, in every country, following the examples of the United States and of Belgium. May the books in this series—and this one in particular—bring that day nearer.

It is necessary—alas—before concluding this preface to inform the reader that he cannot now go to Vienna to verify Mlle. Ganz's observations (nor those of another writer in the present series, M. Dottrens[1]).

There are no more experimental schools in Vienna, neither Adlerian nor any others. The Austrian school is being wholly transformed by an attempt to align it with the new principles of State which impose the confessional idea and that of patriotism as the exclusive inspirations of education and culture. Many innovations dating from the scholastic reforms of 1919 and 1920 have been abandoned because they have been found—or are believed—to contradict this new political orientation. For this, as usual, present financial distress is also alleged, though that argument is feeble to anyone who remembers the state of the Austrian finances at the very time when Glöckel and Fadrus brought about an almost miraculous reform.

Let us not, however, paint the picture too black. The bell has been rung to reverse engines, but the teachers are not

[1] Robert Dottrens, *L'education nouvelle en Autriche*, also published in the *Collection d'Actualités Pédagogiques.*

xiv

all showing much alacrity to go backwards. Many principles of the progressive school are yet in force. It is decreed that schools must give up the reading of complete works and return to the use of 'reading-books', but no such book has yet been published. Still, Vienna to-day is no longer, in this matter of schooling, the place that M. Dottrens and Mlle. Ganz have described, and we owe it to the reader to say so.

The storm has laid low many a tree that was in splendid bloom and able to bear rich fruit. Will these ever flourish again in the ground where they were first planted? To the great friends of children whose names we have recalled, we wish it with full hearts. But we are glad to know that, whatever may happen, the seeds of their planting are now being sown to the winds of the world, and that this book, too, will contribute to their dissemination.

Geneva   PIERRE BOVET

Translator's Note

ADLER's Individual Psychology is not a new subject, nor is this a new book about it; it is the translation of a treatise written as long ago as 1935. Both before that date and after it, books written in, or translated into, English have enriched our knowledge of Alfred Adler and of his contribution to the revolution in psychology.[1] What has still been lacking, however, is an eye-witness's account of the Adlerian psychology in action in the social surroundings out of which it arose. That is what Dr. Schmid-Ganz's book so admirably supplies.

Of the great Viennese psychiatrists Alfred Adler was unquestionably the one who looked, worked and lived most like the family doctor in his 'pastoral' function. He was also, by his social—and to a lesser extent political—sympathies a socialist; his psychology is essentially directed towards the reconciliation of the individual with society. Like Freud and his colleagues, whose debates he frequented in the early 1900's, Adler had to deal with the psychoneuroses that were rife in Vienna during its decline and still more so after its fall from imperial power. It was primarily from the treatment of adult patients, mostly of the middle and upper classes, that he acquired his psychological knowledge. But the normative principle of his 'Individual Psychology' was the *sense of the community*, and he early sought to have his therapeutic methods used more widely in the educational and psychosocial problems of his native city. In that epoch, which might well be called the psychological Enlighten-

[1] For recent examples, see Phyllis Bottome's biographical study *Alfred Adler, Apostle of Freedom* (Faber & Faber, 1939) and Lewis Way's *Adler's Place in Psychology* (Allen & Unwin, 1950).

ment, it was Alfred Adler and his disciples who, more than any others, applied themselves systematically to the problems of the teachers and parents of primary schoolchildren.

The value of the Adlerian methodology is therefore not to be found only by theoretical comparison (important though that may be) with the doctrines of his great contemporaries. Nor is it proved by the wide currency that his ideas so quickly gained in Europe and America, nor even, perhaps, is it to be seen in the consulting rooms of the many psychiatrists who have learned from his methods and practise them with success. The value and validity of Adler's standpoint was best demonstrated by the teachers, physicians and psychiatrists whom he inspired to work in the shabby purlieus of the stricken metropolis—the devoted 'field-workers' whose labours are movingly recorded here by Dr. Schmid-Ganz.

Adler's name would not be written indelibly as it is, among those of the creators of the new depth-psychology, if the social insight which was his essential contribution had not found expression in such action. This school of psychotherapy could not have consistently confined itself to the prolonged and expensive treatment of individual sufferers from social decadence. The work that these devotees did in the Viennese schools was part and parcel of their whole psychological outlook, and Adler continued to promote and sustain their efforts until he was finally exiled by the political troubles that followed upon the rise of National Socialism over the German border.

Adler's work as a whole has been relatively underrated in recent years, and this particular expression of his ideas was never the most widely publicized. While the literature of Adlerian theory spread swiftly abroad, it was natural that the widest currency was obtained for what was most useful in private practice, or most attractive to general readers interested either academically or because of their own psychic problems. To some, the educational work savoured too much of something like philanthropic or missionary effort; and indeed it had to be carried on at sacrifice and was rarely profitable to write about by those engaged in it. The *International Zeitschrift für Individual Psychologie* was their professional organ, published only in German, and was all they had time for. It is fortunate that Dr. Schmid-Ganz was enabled to live for a while in Vienna expressly to produce the following study.

The outline of Adlerian principles with which she begins is as clear and comprehensive as any equally brief exposition available. Nor does it 'date' seriously, for Adler's death, followed so soon by the dispersal of his disciples and the disruptions of the war, inhibited further development of Adlerianism as a school of thought. Elaborations and refinements of principle and practice have been made by individual Adlerians, but these do not invalidate anything in Dr. Schmid-Ganz's summary, which gives the best possible idea of what was in the minds of those engaged in the activities she records. It also presents very effectively 'what every teacher ought to know' about Adler's contribution to education.

The translation of this book has been a congenial task for one who enjoyed for a time the great privilege of personal co-operation with Alfred Adler in his work. I am glad to be able thus to acknowledge the enduring debt that I owe in common with so many others for the humanity and stoicism of his example as well as for the wisdom of his teaching which seemed to alter one's entire relation to life. This book has many times turned my imagination back to the few days in Vienna where I saw the sage in action, as a lecturer and physician, at leisure in his house and garden at Suleymansdorf, and in conversation with his colleagues and disciples talking far into the night at the Café Siller. These are such memories as one would in any case recall from time to time with affection. But recollections of another kind, less likely to recur spontaneously, are no less vividly called up by this book—those of a late afternoon, in a bleak schoolroom in a poor quarter of the city, where one was privileged to be present at the proceedings of one of those psycho-pedagogic councils which furnished the main material of the present treatise. It was a moving as well as most instructive experience only to look on at such colloquies between mother and child, doctor and teacher, carried on generally with such tact and candour and transparent naturalness.

Whether anything resembling these advisory councils could or should be instituted elsewhere is a question for those more competent to answer it. These institutions arose in an urban society with its own unique characteristics, in a certain prolonged crisis of its history. They were suspended during a phase of further social destruction, and had no conspicuous place in the post-war reorganization of education in Vienna But Dr. Oskar Spiel, mentioned in this book, is head of a high school there, working in the same spirit and tradition. And that there is a revival of Adlerian practice is shown by the reappearance of the *Zeitschrift*.

Dr. Schmid-Ganz's treatise is of an interest beyond that of its psychological content: to the sociologist it represents the effort of a highly civilized society to cope with forces of disintegration that threatened the intimate structure of its biological life, a response to one of the challenges of history. The Austrian metropolis is not the only one that is thus menaced now after a second world war. For this reason also, sociologists as well as teachers will be glad to have access to the data that this author has put on record.

Foreword

Our residence in Vienna during the winter of 1932–3 has enabled us to record our personal experience of an inestimable work which a few persons, heroically devoted to their vocation as educators, have accomplished in conditions of dire poverty. It is our heartfelt desire to make this known to all whose lives bring them into daily contact with children—with those little people who depend so much upon us to-day, but who to-morrow will be the managers of the world.

Day after day we followed the course of instruction in the remarkable experimental school of Adlerian pedagogy, collecting as much documentation about it as we could, and never failing to amplify our own observations with the invaluable information that the teachers were so willing to impart. It gives us the greatest pleasure here to express our warm gratitude for this to Drs. Spiel, Birnbaum, and Scharmer, the devoted triumvirate who were the life and soul of that school.

The better to estimate the work this school was doing, we also visited about sixty classes in the ordinary public schools, receiving everywhere, we are happy to acknowledge, the same benevolent courtesy.

It should be said in advance that our participation in the proceedings of the medico-pedagogic councils differed a good deal under the different directors who presided over them. Sometimes we were only listeners taking shorthand notes, whilst in other instances we ourselves took part in conversations with the parents and with the children. We were then privileged to share the invaluable experience of direct personal contact with the individuals, more or less unstable, who came to ask for advice. At other times, moreover, where a case needed to be studied and influenced in its own surroundings, we were entrusted with the task of visiting a child regularly at its home.

Thanks to the Adlerian doctors and advisers, who with such great geniality initiated us into their pioneer work, we were able to supplement our observations by those which had been made before our stay in Vienna. Mesdames Lehndorff, Löwy, Deutsch, Holub, Seidler, Lazarsfeld, Friedmann, as well as Mm. Wexberg, Deutsch, Krauss and Zanker, by whose generosity we were enabled to collect the necessary material, are entitled to all our gratitude for this. Nor do we forget, after having been received with such cordiality by the Viennese psychologists and teachers, who rightly profess their keen admiration for the Institute of Science and Education, that we owe it also to the kindness of Professor Pierre Bovet. This adds to our pleasure in recording here our feelings of profound thankfulness for the advice and encouragement he has so often and abundantly supplied.

Dr. Adler himself, who, since his appointment to Long Island Medical College at New York, was no longer available for regular consultation, willingly placed at our disposal the records kept for several years, and from these we have taken the cases described on pages 152, 162, 164. To Dr. Adler we owe all the devotion of a disciple to the master who has shown him the right way, and we heartily wish, for the work of so great and so modest a man, an ever-widening influence. May his noble example be followed by the steadily-growing number of those who understand that psychological harmony—to which humanity has so long aspired—can be realized only in the creative synthesis of individual and social strivings. If this small book succeeds in awakening, among the French-speaking public, wider interest in this great Viennese psychologist and educator and in his remarkable achievement, it will have fully attained the end at which it aims.

Historical Introduction

NOTIONS expressing some kind of knowledge of the human soul are found among all peoples in every age; and in this sense 'psychology' can be said to be as old as mankind. But whilst this knowledge formerly constituted only a branch of philosophy and was practised only intuitively, the nineteenth century turned it into an independent science with the discipline of a methodical acquisition of knowledge. Only then did psychology pass from the pre-scientific stage to that of a science properly so called. What was it made this development possible? It was thanks to psychotherapy. It was the study of innumerable cases of human suffering which led to the analysis and understanding, in their complexity, of the factors which make up the existing personality of man.

We shall not linger here to recall the decisive influences exercised by such men as Charcot, Bernheim, Janet and Breuer. For the same reason the illuminating theories of Sigmund Freud will be taken as read. It is with the latter that the *individual psychology* of Alfred Adler, itself a product of psychopathology, is connected historically. But Adler, who was at the same time a medical practitioner and a psychologist, developed a psychotherapy into what was also an educational method of the highest importance.

For several years, from 1902 to 1908, Adler was a disciple and collaborator of Freud, though he never entered into close personal relations with the man whose immense services to psychology he so profoundly esteemed. And as his own fundamental conceptions (concerning the neuroses, sexuality, heredity and the relation between prior and final causes) carried him further and further away from those of Freud, Adler was not slow to draw the natural consequences. In 1912, in the Society for Individual Psychology (*Verein für Individualpsychologie*) he paved the way for a new orientation of research. From that time onward Adlerian psychology is clearly distinguished from the stream of psychoanalysis.

If it be true, then, that Adler found his point of departure with Freud, he was soon to part company with his master. The divergences between the two systems are well known. Far from setting up sexuality as the main principle of interpretation, as Freud had done, Adler relegated it to an importance secondary to that of the *will to power* (*Machtstreben*). That is the opposition which is obvious at a first reading. Upon a deeper comparison, one observes that the Freudian theory is essentially preoccupied with the past, that it explains the integral reality analytically, in terms of cause and effect, to the exclusion of all freedom and spontaneous creation. That is the root of its pessimism. Adler, on the other hand, continually directs our vision towards 'the land of our children'—to borrow a phrase from Nietzsche. For him, efficient causes explain but one aspect of the reality; and he adduces the notion of 'final causality' as the only one that enables us to render an account of life, of being and becoming. His conception of 'productive action', of the free development of the personality in striving towards a higher goal, is the source of all Adler's optimism. His conception of man as a totality, with an immanent teleology, relates him to the German psychologists E. Spranger and W. Stern.

CHAPTER ONE

The Theory of Adlerian Psychology

A. WHAT IS ALFRED ADLER'S PSYCHOLOGY?

BEFORE attempting a theoretical exposition of Adlerian psychology, it is advisable to emphasize certain necessary distinctions. From the *formal* point of view, then, we distinguish, on the one hand, the psychology of the whole from a symptomatology of its various parts considered separately; and on the other hand we distinguish between finalistic explanations and causal explanations.

From the *material* point of view, namely from that of content, Adlerian psychology takes account of everything that concerns the individual, society and their mutual relations. Although all these factors obviously interpenetrate in actuality, their analysis is indispensable in theory if we are to acquire an adequate knowledge of any individual.

1. *A psychology of totality*

The German word itself — 'Individualpsychologie' — easily gives rise to a misunderstanding, for one is tempted to think it means a psychology that applies to the individual exclusively. But if one refers to the etymological sense of the word (*individere*) its field of application is much more extensive. This is the psychology of 'the whole that cannot be divided' concerned at one and the same time with the individual as he is in himself and in his relation to the community. Just as medicine is no longer—as a general rule—satisfied with the separate treatment of morbid symptoms, but proceeds to take account of the condition of the entire organism, neither should psychology be limited to

3

the study of certain phenomena in isolation from the psyche as a whole.

In the totality of its organic and psychic functions the individual constitutes an original unity, which it expresses at every moment through all its movements internal and external. But this unity is in its turn but a part of the higher unity constituted by society. This conception of 'totality' is not wholly new, since one finds it, or at least a more or less marked tendency towards it, in many modern psychologists, notably Spranger and Stern. What is however genuinely characteristic of Adlerian psychology is the linking of this conception with that of an immanent finalism.

2. A psychology of finality

The principle of the efficient cause, productive as it is in the realm of material science, is inadequate in that of psychology. Adlerian psychology therefore appeals beyond this to the final cause. For instance, if a child does not tell the truth, one does not ask only, 'what causes it to lie' but equally, 'what is the aim it has in view'. For everything that an individual does, it does in order to attain a goal that it sets itself, consciously or unconsciously.

These two conceptions of the cause, far from being mutually exclusive, are moreover complementary, since the reality as a whole consists in the close interpenetration of the efficient cause and the final cause.

By taking the principle of finality into consideration, the Adlerian psychology has an advantage over any psychology that admits only efficient causes. Such exclusiveness leads inevitably to rigorous determinism and ultimate pessimism. The intervention of finality, on the other hand, enables the Adlerian to extend the view into the future, with a palpable gain in optimism. The past (which plays the essential part in efficient causal explanation) is allowed only so much attention as is necessary in order to overcome it. The present situation is the point of departure, but the goal is a better future. The past is made to serve simply as a means of finding out the *style of life* that the individual is always and everywhere pursuing, and that only to assist in his education or re-education.

The finality of the personality is manifested in all the actions of an individual, even in those which at first sight appear the least significant—in forgetting, for example; one repeatedly forgets intentions or facts if they are embarrassing. The same observation can be made about *remembering*, for one remembers most easily whatever contributes to the attainment of one's goal. With this in view, the interpretation of *dreams* can furnish us with useful indications. Unlike Freud, who attributes to dreams a language whose symbols need only to be translated into other terms (from the 'manifest content' to the 'latent content') Adler lays down no rules, for he does not consider the dream interpretable except as a function of the whole personality: for him the dream is but one of the innumerable manifestations of the individual. It anticipates the future, constituting a 'probeweiser Anschlag'—which may be translated as a 'trial project'. Disencumbered of all logical calculation, the individual gives free rein to his feelings; he 'tries out' a realization of his hopes, or a resolution of the conflicts he suffers in the waking state. He puts himself into the mood (Stimmung) which will dominate his behaviour on the morrow.

B. DEFINITION OF SOME FUNDAMENTAL CONCEPTS

Certain concepts play a fundamental part in the psychology of Adler:

1. *The feeling of inferiority* (*Minderwertigkeitsgefühl*)

Does this feeling exist in every individual? Adlerian psychology replies in the affirmative, with the reservation that the feeling may be more or less marked or more or less compensated according to the individual's self-development. From the moment at which the baby discovers its *self*, when it understands, for instance, that its foot is a portion of itself, its desires outstrip the possibility of their realization, the latter being dependent upon physical growth. In the course of its first fumblings the infant finds itself deserted, and is bound to suffer from a sense of abandonment. When it discovers the 'other' it will be consoled by the evidence that other beings like itself exist. But since these others—usually the parents, or older brothers and sisters—are adults who are apparently omnipotent and omniscient, the infant cannot but feel at the same time its weakness and dependence. These first experiences of weakness and dependence are the origin of the 'feeling of inferiority'. This however we cannot verify directly. What we observe is, on the contrary, a striving towards power, superiority or perfection (Geltungsstreben). The infant tries to surpass its actual condition; it shows a tendency to make itself felt, to be more than it is. We can interpret this ambition as a compensation for its feeling of inferiority, an hypothesis we adopt because it enables us to demonstrate the finality in infantile behaviour with satisfactory results. *Inferiority-feeling* and the *striving for power* constitute, as it were, the negative and positive poles of the same current of development, each equally indispensable to the growth of the infant; and so long as they remain in reasonable equilibrium they guarantee its normal development. It is the tension between these opposites that sustains the tone and feeling of personality, without which no one can become a useful member of the community.

The last factor to be mentioned, one that is often determinative of the inferiority-feeling, is organic inferiority. All the organs of our body have their appropriate functions, and an ill-developed or atrophied organ is felt by the individual as an inferiority. Such ill-developed organs constitute *loci minoris resistentiae*—i.e., they can easily become the seat of the most diverse maladies. We find that these blemishes are as likely to occur in the respiratory or digestive tracts, in the uro-genital system, in the circulatory or nervous systems, or in the glands of internal secretion, as in the organs of the higher senses, the eyes or the ears; and such organic inferiorities are generally compensated by the heightened activity of another organ. The classic example in medicine is that of the removal of one kidney which provokes an additional activity of the other. Similar compensations can arise in the sphere of the psyche. The defective organ occasions an accentuation of the individual's energies as a whole, a fact which explains why there are so many musicians with defective hearing and so many painters who suffer from visual abnormalities. In these cases it is not a matter of compensation but of *over-compensation*, for the individual is stimulated to do something more than he would if the organ in question were normal. Let us note here a significant fact indicated for the first time by Adlerian psychologists—that the same organic inadequacies produce entirely different consequences in different individuals, because everything here depends upon the kind of importance that the subject attaches to his specific disability. A man with weak vision can become a shirker, excusing himself before society and to himself by saying that 'if he had normal sight he would have been an excellent painter'. Another man in the same situation will, on the contrary, concentrate all his energies precisely upon painting, and perhaps succeed in producing some remarkable works. We know that Beethoven was deaf when he produced his most grandiose work the ninth symphony. There is abundant proof that the compensation of an organic inferiority depends less upon the actual handicap it imposes than upon the manner in which the suffering individual reacts to it. Everything depends finally upon the attitude he assumes towards his physical constitution. The more courageous this is, the less pronounced will be his feeling of inferiority, and the better his general performance.

2. *The feeling of community* (*Gemeinschaftsgefühl*)

From the feeling of inferiority we are led directly to the feeling of community. For the more the subject suffers from the feeling of inferiority the less capable he is of any genuine co-operation; and, conversely, such capacity for co-operation as he has increases proportionately as the individual gains confidence in his own powers. The two kinds of feeling develop, so to speak, in inverse ratio one with another.

The individual abandoned wholly to himself would be unable to survive. It was in order not to perish that man became a social being. At the present day, this characteristic of sociability may be regarded as innate, and it is according to the degree of its development in the child that he acquires the *feeling of community* in Adler's sense. Adler regards this as something of a higher order than the social instinct properly so called. It is not, like the latter, satisfied by the common life in a society constituted by a mere multiplicity of individuals. It sets up an ideal demand, the aspiration for a community towards which one ought to strive continually, though it may never be actually attained. It is made up of sympathy and love for one's fellows, not merely arising out of common interest but also, *sub specie aeternitatis*, out of objectivity in face of realities, devotion and

8

responsibility. It is from his community-feeling that man acknowledges his membership of this great organism the Universe, and upon the development of this feeling depend all the values that he is capable of creating.

The feeling of community implies the acceptance of the three fundamental tasks enumerated by Adler:

The duty of attaining competence in some occupation

This is seen less from the moral than from the rational point of view, since a faulty performance of this task will be injurious both to the individual and to society.

The duty of goodwill towards one's fellows (Mitmenschlichkeit)

This duty is incumbent in the first place upon the family, since the interest that the child will take in other people is conditioned by the confidence he acquires in his own powers. By virtue of the principle of reciprocity, the individual who avoids all contact with others will soon find himself let well alone, while he who treats the others with confidence will soon be surrounded with genuine friends. Wexberg is right in saying that it is easier to love 'the whole world' than to dwell in perfect community with a few friends.

The duty towards the opposite sex

Every relationship founded upon love necessarily imposes upon either party its share of responsibility. No sound relationship is possible without a courageous affirmation, which implies the joyful acceptance of this responsibility.

Here as elsewhere, and perhaps with more difficulty than elsewhere, only the frank and courageous individual will succeed.

3. *The concept of heredity*

Here we touch upon a question that is still very controversial. Its importance in relation to Adlerian psychology is in estimating how far a man's manner of acting is determined by hereditary factors. Certain hereditary blemishes in the form and the functioning of certain organs are admitted, in, for example, cases of syphilitic or alcoholic ancestry. But in regard to this Adler makes a point of capital importance; namely that the defect of an organ, whether of its form or function, never determines in advance the use which its possessor will make of it. He goes so far as to say: 'It matters little what we bring with us into the world, everything depends upon what we do with it.' This view recalls that of Claparède, in whose opinion no one can change his 'mental equipment' but only the way he avails himself of it.

The question before us is, then, to what extent we are capable of overcoming hereditary defects.

One can see at once that the answer must vary according to the nature of the defect; it is obvious that a blind man, for example, cannot make himself into a painter. But nothing prevents his becoming a musician if he wishes to devote himself to music. Or, to take the case of a complete weakling, clearly incapable of an intellectual career or perhaps of embracing any profession at all, there is no proof that the fundamental disabilities under which he labours will make a criminal of him. In spite of all, education can and ought to turn this disinherited person into a social being; for it is the formidable task of education to render everyone, whatever he may be, valuable to the community. To this end, education needs to be able to initiate every individual into his best way of living, taking into account his particular physical and psychic constitution.

Adlerian psychology in no wise neglects the problems of heredity. On the contrary, while admitting its inability to resolve them theoretically in the present state of science, it adduces practical solutions. These invariably consist in seeking how to make the best of what is at the individual's disposal. What is the best course to take, in the given case, in order to obtain the most socially-favourable result?

In the Adlerian view, all the responsibility for ultimate success or failure devolves upon education, first upon that of the family and the school, and then upon the subject's self-education. For what is decisive, in this view, is the attitude that the individual assumes towards what life has given him, and that attitude is educable. All the optimism of Adler resides in this affirmation.

Moreover, he has frequently been able to demonstrate that backward children, believed for that reason to have been suffering from hereditary defects, were in fact the victims of discouragement due to the educational deficiency or incompetence of their environment. Have we not ourselves discovered often enough that the retarded development of a child has been considerably compensated by a more appropriate training, conducted with perseverance? However cautious one may be about prejudging such an issue, one has to recognize that no sharp distinction can ever be drawn between the products of heredity and those of education; and since the possibilities of education seem to be practically unlimited, Adlerian psychology is justified in overstepping any bounds imposed only by theories as yet unverified. So long as science can prove nothing to the contrary, it is permissible to think we can best deal with hereditary factors by ameliorating others that are accessible —that is, those of the family and the school. In medicine, a parallel case, the practitioner has no time to wait for the definitive findings of scientific researches: he has to act immediately, upon the knowledge immediately at his disposal. Similarly, in pedagogy, practice is obliged to go beyond current theory.

It is appropriate at this point to say a word about capabilities (Begabung). Not infrequently one has the surprise of finding, upon closer knowledge of a person who is regarded as gifted in one way or another, that his capability is the result of a compensation. It was originally an inferiority which, followed by an intensive training, has produced a performance well above the average.

During the development of an individual, an appropriate training may lead to the sudden appearance of an aptitude hitherto ignored; and conversely, a discouragement can bring about the disappearance, sometimes finally, of qualities that were formerly exceptional. We shall see later on, in the chapter upon the Adlerian experimental school, how much of the aptitudes that the children display depends upon the qualities of the teacher. Nor must one disregard the fact that a child may be trying to draw profit from its attendance at school in order to realize a style of life outside the community. This means that one must be able to distinguish between *the child who is willing but cannot* and *the child who can, but does not want to.*

A child that had long been considered incapable of arithmetic, has suddenly, under a new teacher, found itself among the first in that subject. Since we must dismiss the idea that aptitudes can appear and disappear in a purely arbitrary fashion, we must prefer the explanation offered by Adlerian psychology, which, as we have seen, ascribes such a change to courage and training, while fully admitting the secondary influence of certain innate factors.

In short, primary importance must be attributed to the physical condition of the given individual, to the surroundings in which he lives, and to the greater or lesser degree of courage he brings to the making of the best possible use of his condition.

C. ENVIRONMENTAL INFLUENCES

1. The family

The social environment is constituted by a complexity of influences. First and foremost, for the child of either sex, is that of the mother; it is she who satisfies its needs in earliest infancy and is the first object of its desires. When a perfect relation is established between mother and infant child, it is a sure guarantee that the latter will act with confidence in later life. But once this relation is secured, the next duty of the mother is to see that it does not become exclusive, but to direct the infant's interest towards the father and towards any brothers and sisters that there may be. In the course of forming these relations one after another the sense of community is awakened in the child; and it is then that the *father* ought to continue its education, enabling it to pass beyond the familial nest into the world at large.

The motherless orphan is thus liable to suffer from lack of confidence, and its feeling for community is often ill-developed; that is, it shows a tendency to timidity and unsociability. As for the child deprived of a father, the danger is that without his living example it may never grasp the meaning of work and the obligation to win a livelihood, which will give it greater difficulties than most children have in finding their place in the bosom of the community.

Adlerian psychology also places great emphasis upon the place of the child within its family. Is it an only boy or girl? Or, if there are brothers and sisters, what is its place in the order of succession?

These are questions that have their importance. The only child, for instance, is very generally a 'spoiled' child. Those around it endeavour to smooth every obstacle from its path; they exert themselves to gratify its every whim; and when a child of such an upbringing comes to school, wholly unarmed to meet the difficulties it must now encounter, it will commonly develop nervous symptoms. It may weep, or wet its bed at night, but the precise symptom is, in this connexion, of little importance. In order to hold in school the exceptional position that it occupied at home, such a child may strive to attain it by attracting the attention of others—by grimaces, for example, or by any attitude that upsets the discipline of the class. When he is older, he will always be eager to play some part out of the ordinary. But as such an individual will be almost always incapable of doing this to any genuine purpose, he will try to content himself by being *unique* in some sphere merely accessory or useless to society, if not actually harmful.

Or consider the case of the pampered child whom its parents one day present with a brother or sister. It may very well happen that this child suffers cruelly by having to share the solicitude which had hitherto been its sole privilege; and the event may fill it with a bitterness that underlies all its subsequent life.

Different ways of development may be open to the eldest child of the family. In the best case, it will develop well, and soon set an example to its brothers and sisters. But if it also suffers from the feeling that more is demanded of it than it has to give, it will gradually become timid and discouraged. This will incline it to harbour feelings of culpability, or unhealthy ambition, which may check every impulse to work as soon as it arises. A boy will perhaps assert himself as a veritable tyrant over his brothers and sisters; lacking confidence in himself, he will try at least to appear forceful in the eyes of others.

In second sons one often observes two opposite attitudes. The one consists in giving up the struggle from the beginning, because to such children it seems impossible ever to equal their older brothers and sisters: the other tends to safeguard its prestige in spite of everything, by asserting this in a realm where no one will be able to assail it. There are cases in which we see children taking a line entirely apart from their family, thereby rendering any comparison with the others impossible. These are the revolutionaries, often souls who nourish inordinate ambitions.

As to the children whose destiny has placed them in the midst of several brothers and sisters, they are the privileged ones from this point of view of the *family constellation*. For it should not be difficult for them to serve as examples to the younger ones while themselves benefiting from those of their elders.

We cannot here attempt to give an exhaustive account of the possibilities of the *family constellation*, but can only offer some general observations. For example, a child that is a very late-comer after a numerous family may play a part in it similar to that of an only son or daughter.

It is important to know the position that a child occupies in the family, for to know this always enables the teacher to draw valuable inferences. This position, as we have seen, can often provide advantage as well as disadvantage for the child, since in the final reckoning everything depends upon its own reaction. To be informed of this circumstance enables the educator to co-operate beneficially.

It is no exaggeration to say that a good family training is an advantage that affects the entire subsequent life of an individual. One should never seek to replace it by institutional care, conferred outside the family, except in cases where the atmosphere is definitely malefic. In that case, indeed, an institutional upbringing is the lesser of two evils. But for the child nothing, we repeat, can ever fully replace the education it can receive from a father and mother aware of their responsibility.

2. *Different educational methods*

Unfortunately it must be recognized that the educator's responsibilities are often ill-understood. Let us consider briefly the well-known *firm* or *authoritative* method, with its ideal of the model child. The ideal being of necessity chimerical, this method can in fact succeed only in producing an atrophied child, accustomed to incessant compliance and incapable of initiative; or else a shut-up individual, living in constant opposition to the authority that seeks its subjection, and striving to circumvent it by innumerable subterfuges. When it is required to accomplish anything that demands frankness and energy, a child brought up on the 'firm method' will almost invariably show incapacity.

The majority of children subjected to authoritarian education choose the convenient path of *deviation*. Believing, from their education, that they are weak and inferior, they struggle to produce, in themselves and before others, proof to the contrary. Thus they may often become heroes of a kind but in, so to speak, a negative direction. In the better cases, which are rare (Adlerian psychology does not even mention them) the child is pliant just as long as authority makes itself felt, and recovers its force and assurance as soon as authority is withdrawn. But in such a case there is always reason to ask oneself 'What might not this child have become, had it only been fully and properly educated?'

We shall say but a few words about *religious* education, if only because this seems to be growing steadily more uncommon. Such education is often excellent in itself, provided that the child is made to feel that its parents truly acknowledge a divine principle over themselves: but it is dangerous when parents use it only as a means of strengthening their own authority. That kind of profanation of the name of God is not so rare as one would like to believe, and such admonitions as these—'If you are not good, God will punish you' or 'If you tell me a lie, God will tell me about it', have come to the ears of most of us. The effects of such treatment can be disastrous, for it tends more or less rapidly to extinguish all the child's respect and admiration for what is beyond and above it.

Beside the parents who adopt these more or less definite educational methods there is the whole range of those who bring up their children without well knowing how or, as one might say, by guess-work.

Many children are reared without affection by parents who readily lift their hand against them. Understandably enough they become mistrustful, unable to fulfil the duties that the community has a right to expect from them and without regard for their equals. Others are subjected to an education far too ambitious on the part of their parents, because the latter are eager, at any price, to see their progeny successful in something they were unable to do themselves. Such education is not without danger, because too tense an atmosphere is plainly unfavourable to a child's development, apart from the fact that the least set-back will be taken as a catastrophe. One must not forget, however, that the trespasses committed against the child proceed less, in an Adlerian view, from the educational method itself than from the parents' mistaken ways of living. Example is the most effective of teachers, and it is the way in which the parents live—irrespective of their good or bad ideas about education—that invariably plays the principal part. This one must be careful not to underestimate; but one must not therefore neglect the simultaneous education of the educators, by showing them, for example, when their authoritarian procedure is prompted by a wish to compensate for their own inferiority-feeling, etc.

3. *The economic situation*

The social class, and the material circumstances of the family, are factors that influence the child from birth. One is tempted to affirm that a good education is possible whatever the social and material situation of the family may be, and in reality so it is. For though these circumstances themselves, when they are adverse, obviously increase educational difficulties, the decisive influence they too often have proceeds, in most cases, from the exaggerated importance that is attached to them.

For convenience, we will distinguish the social class of those who possess practically nothing, living from day to day by their employment when they have any, from the class of the bourgeois and that of the rich. These categories signify very little to-day, since profound transformations in most of our countries have overturned the established positions of pecuniary advantage, and in reality the overwhelming majority are now practically without property. The term 'class' in this sense is justified only because certain ways of living corresponding to property-positions have survived their disappearance.

It remains true that the children born into a very poor family suffer above all in their physical development, from insufficiency both of nourishment and of necessary care. Moreover, the monotony and often the misery of such a situation soon make their consequences felt in the most troublesome ways. Totally deprived of pleasures, children in this position generally nurse an almost unbelievable longing for money and luxuries. From this they are led, little by little, to form a most depressing conception of life, a stark materialism in which the supreme good is the possession of as much money as possible. To children growing up in such privation, the acquisition of a fortune seems to be the only ideal of any real interest. Would not a fortune enable them to procure everything they see other people enjoying—every comfort and delight? It is very understandable that money should become the one great preoccupation of those to whom life has shown itself so miserly.

In the great towns, many young children are left almost completely to their own devices, either from lack of hearth and home, or because 'home' is a theatre for such violent scenes that they occupy it as little as possible. These are the unfortunate ones who are tempted, when they grow older, to seek refuge and forgetfulness of their misery in drink, which will be their doom after a progressive loss of all human dignity. Some will come at last to the criminal court of which poverty is all too often the antechamber. Indeed the criminal is commonly an individual thirsting for the enjoyments that he feels life has denied him and now set upon attaining them by means injurious to society. As for the girls, they become an easy prey for prostitution, in which they expect to find a simple way of escape from their privations.

In the majority of these cases we have to do with discouraged individuals, who feel themselves to be inferior, frustrated of what ought to be theirs by right, and who are seeking by no matter what means to lift themselves up out of their circumstances. They are of course choosing the wrong way and deceiving themselves, for it leads to no betterment of their condition, but the very reverse.

At the opposite end of the social scale are the rich, for whom the problem would appear much simpler, since they have ample means at disposal to provide their children with the best possible education. In reality their advantage is not nearly so great as it looks. For the rich are very commonly unprepared to resist the lures of luxury: they too often spoil their children, who are thus ill-prepared for life and in danger of growing up weak and emasculated.

It is in the so-called bourgeois class, as a general rule, that we find the best conditions for a good education. Their state of life, in which the mother gives a great deal of attention to her children, represents the golden mean between insufficiency and superabundance. Here we find, normally, an atmosphere of frankness and tranquillity, but also of activity, in which the child can develop its sense of community without set-backs. Danger—for obviously that exists everywhere—may lurk in the excessive ambition entertained by some parents on behalf of their children: but we will not elaborate this point, which we have already touched upon in regard to different educational methods.

One may believe, or at least hope, that these remarks upon the economic factor in education will at no distant date be unrelated to realities. For this, however, we must await the triumph of that movement towards greater social justice which is a hopeful sign of our times.

D. THE STYLE OF LIFE OR THE PLAN OF LIFE
(*Lebensstil, Leitlinie*)

To form a correct conception of any individual, we have to note his behaviour towards others, his *capacity for contact* (Kontaktfähigkeit). In Adlerian terms, to get to know anyone is to *perceive his style of life*. For every 'self' is subject to its own *individual law of movement*. This law is decreed by heredity (in the measure previously indicated), by the influences of the environment and, finally, by the existing polarity between the feeling of inferiority and the striving for power (Machtstreben). The sum of these different factors constitutes what is called the *psychic constitution* of the individual. Hence this constitution is acquired, unlike the physical constitution which is almost always innate. This means that the psychic constitution is not determined in any rigorous sense, as people are often inclined to believe (generally, however, in order to excuse the mediocrity of their performance!). For two at least of the three factors that combine to form the style of life are modifiable: the environmental influences and the feeling of inferiority, both susceptible of *compensation*. Thanks to this psychological insight, radical reorientation of character has become possible for anyone who has grasped the educability of these factors, which formerly seemed inaccessible to any influence.

The style of life, which is manifested at every instant by our behaviour, is subject to the law of finality. In the most diverse circumstances, and generally without his being aware of it, the individual is working towards an *end*. This may be, for instance, to occupy an extraordinary position; or, by an appearance of timidity in the eyes of others to attract their interest and support. To this end a child may work badly or not at all at school, or disturb the class by every sort of stupidity, for the sole reason that it unconsciously desires to realize this aim—to focus upon itself the attention of its master and classmates. As Adler shows, every normal individual has a plan of life, only the feeble-minded and the abnormal are without one. That is the one distinction he would draw between normality and abnormality in children, for any other line we try to draw between them inevitably fluctuates.

For the formation of its plan (or style) of life, which is a creative act, the material is given to the child. And as we have seen, this material counts for less than the attitude assumed towards it. For Adlerian psychology, one's successes and failures result primarily from one's goal, according to whether this is shaped in accord or disaccord with the logic of life. His own researches have led Adler to the conclusion that the style of life is generally formed during the first five years of childhood. From that time onward every action and every thought of the individual will follow the line of direction already established. In cases where a radical alteration becomes necessary, it is possible only if the individual attains to a truer knowledge of himself. He must understand the error he made in the fixation of his goal, and change the standpoint from which all his actions have been seen by himself in an entirely false perspective. Then, but only then, a re-education based upon his new insight into himself will be possible.

As we have seen, the problems which present themselves to every one of us at one time or another can all be referred to one of three categories: those of society, profession or the sexual relation. To the resolution of these problems, every one applies himself in a different way, according to his or her 'individual law'. Adler distinguishes four kinds of inadequate 'movement' among persons who have not sufficiently developed their communal feeling.

1. *The hesitant movement* (die zögernde Bewegung)

The individual's action is slow, his rhythm is irregular and there is little perseverance. Such an individual may be capable of tackling a task with impetuosity, but only to stall completely at the first obstacle. In his general behaviour he shows very little self-confidence.

2. *Distance-keeping*

The individual always keeps himself at a certain distance from reality. One example cited is that of a person who at twenty years of age still has no friends; who at thirty has not brought himself to embrace any profession, and who, at forty, has never been in love.

3. *The movement of flight*

The individual is always trying to escape from his duty

along some secret path. This is the most common type of abnormal 'movement', for it comprehends every kind of *deviation*.

4. *The partial movement*

The individual cannot bring himself to attack any problem as a whole. He has to divide it into little portions and try to deal with them one after another. This 'piece-meal' movement is seen in many neurotic adults.

To sum up; every action and every gesture of a person derives from its directive line of life, which is usually fixed from about the age of five. This he will pursue until the day when he is forced, by repeated defeats, to acknowledge that a reformation of his way of life has become obligatory. We know that such reformation is possible, to the extent that his style of life derives from factors accessible to educative influence (i.e. from those of his social environment and the feeling of inferiority).

We shall see later how painful a thing it is for anyone to undergo such a transformation; it is like finding oneself suspended in the void, between an old life-style that is vanishing and a new one not yet formed, a nameless terror that makes the subject cling more tightly than ever to the way of life from which he is struggling to get free. It may mobilize all his powers in a last effort of defence, a desperate resort to 'security-measures' (Sicherungen) in order to justify his total failure of courage: that is, he will undertake to prove, to the doctor or the teacher, that in his altogether special case the change is impossible. He will adduce an array of facts and recollections selected from the standpoint of his 'tendencious apperception'. Innumerable arguments will occur to him in demonstration of the impossibility of his re-education, because at the bottom of his heart he prefers his sufferings to a psychic showdown that would compel him to pull down his vanity and give up his false sense of personality. In such a case we have really to deal with an aggression, masked by the methods of the weak, and it is for the skill of the Adlerian doctor or teacher to unravel all these artifices and enable the patient to see them as such. And in so far as the latter himself comes to realize the justice of this demonstration, he will gain in courage and confidence. When his feeling for community grows stronger, he will at last be able to give up his erroneous course of conduct.

One will hardly find in Adlerian terminology such words as right, wrong or culpable in the moral sense. Its interest is directed simply towards right or wrong understanding in decisions for action, as was that of Socrates or of Descartes. But the method is not therefore satisfied with the discernment of error: it holds out hope and assistance to anyone who is too weak to achieve detachment from himself, it can uphold him until an initial success awakens his reliance upon his own strength. By a series of compensations, the individual can then recover his equilibrium, when he will become capable of fulfilling his duties to the community. His style of life will then cease to be, as it were, an automatic arrangement thrown out of gear by the slightest shock, but will assume a dynamic quality, and be able to adapt itself to the everchanging requirements of our continually-moving world.

E. SEXUALITY

To convey what Adler means by the 'masculine protest' (Freud's psychic homosexuality; the 'Diana complex' of Baudouin) a few words must be said about the relative positions of men and women in our culture. Although general opinion upon this subject has changed a good deal in recent years, our society nevertheless remains 'patriarchal' in the sense that the masculine takes precedence over the feminine. This valuation can be seen even in the child: a little girl, as soon as she becomes conscious of her sex, often feels it as an inferiority, and a boy is even more likely to feel pride in the discovery. For him, however, there is also the danger of a haunting fear of losing the supposed 'superiority' (Baudouin's 'castration complex') and it is in that sense that the influence of sexuality may first make itself felt. Conversely, the little girl, if she accepts the assumption that it is 'more worth while' to be a man than a woman, may suddenly take to hoydenish behaviour. She will imitate the boys in every way she can, will take part in their games and exhibit combative instincts. It is this attitude, characteristic of the adolescent girl rebelling against her natural rôle, to which Adler has given the name of 'masculine protest' (Männlicher Protest); an attitude that in certain cases is maintained throughout life. These are the women who strive at any cost to make themselves independent, to become 'emancipated'; who go in for sports, copy masculine attire and habits and sedulously evade the duties of motherhood. In extreme cases, they go so far as the total rejection of their natural rôle, sometimes even turning homosexual. We must observe, however, that such an attitude is often found in women whose natural appearance is not very feminine.

Although the boy, in our climate of thought, enjoys this predominant rôle, it also lays considerable difficulties upon him. He feels he is expected to play the part of a hero and always to make his superiority felt, especially before the girls. To compensate the consequent feelings of inferiority, he may have recourse to physical feats, bullying or boasting: and once puberty is passed he will be tormented by the sexual problem. Yet for lack of confidence in himself he is likely to be afraid of women, and in danger of taking the road that leads to debauchery or to perversion. It is only an harmonious development of feeling, both of his personality and for the community, that really enables a young man to feel confidence with regard to women. For he will then have the strength to give himself without losing himself, and the courage to accept responsibility.

It should be clear, since the sexual problem is but one aspect of the problem of becoming a personality, that sexual education itself can only succeed as part and parcel of this education as a whole.

1. *The perversions*

Masturbation is the commonest form of infantile perversion. There is however no reason to regard it as perverse if we are merely concerned about the practice that is pretty well universal at a certain age. What we have then to deal with is simply a phase to be outgrown, and it will pass without leaving any objectionable traces if the child is growing up under satisfactory conditions.

At its beginning, the child is seeking nothing in masturbation but simple enjoyment. It is only when it has been forbidden to 'amuse itself in that way' that it begins to suffer from a sense of wrongdoing. It is then that a child may acquire the habit of seeking a solace for set-backs in self-gratification (Selbstbefriedigung), and in this way onanism becomes an element of obstinacy. On the other hand, because he suffers, in a struggle which he regards as one between 'good' and 'evil', the masturbator discourages himself more and more, and his feeling of inferiority can grow to the point of completely paralyzing his activity. In order to justify himself in relation to others and in his own eyes, he will take this 'malady' as a fatality that condemns him to a secret life, apart from that of the community.

Infantile masturbation, then, may be no more than a provisional practice and without importance, provided that the educator helps the child to freedom from it, by treating it naturally and encouraging the child while explaining the error of his indulgence. But the habit becomes a perversion when it is practised at an adult age as a substitute for normal sexual behaviour. Here we have to deal with the escape-mechanism of discouraged individuals who are losing self-confidence and becoming incapable of overcoming their fear of women. This is also the case with sadists, masochists and homosexuals, who are always deserters from life, and it is only by an evaluation of their development as a whole that one can hope to understand how they have arrived at such a condition of isolation. Here again, reasoning only from effects to antecedent causes will never bring one to a satisfactory explanation, one has always to reckon with the individual as his own final cause.

2. *The neuroses*

The multiplicity of definitions of neurosis that have been proposed, both from the medical side and from that of psychology both individual and social, only proves how little we yet know about the real nature of this disability. Regarded as an organic illness, psychoneurosis can be plausibly accounted for in terms of causality. But what is new, and characteristic of the Adlerian approach, is to consider it in terms of finality—namely, to ask oneself, with regard to any given case of neurosis, what end might this individual be trying to attain by such behaviour? In most cases the end in view is one of superiority, which he has no courage to seek in the straight, dull ways of the community. And the illness, in which he takes refuge from reality, serves him as an excuse for all that he does not do, or does badly. As Wexberg has said, in an essay upon neurosis,[1] 'Neurosis is a kind of social adaptation (des sozialen Seins), a striving of the individual to affirm himself by means of arrangements and artifices which secure him a permit of freedom from personal responsibility.'

The neurotic symptom thus represents the flight from a decision, due to a sense of inward insecurity. It always indicates some degree of cowardice, for the individual is capitulating in face of the duties that life imposes. The neurotic thinks he will be able to evade the responsibility for his actions by way of the neurosis. His failure of will could be expressed by the formula 'What I would like to do, I cannot do'. He does not grasp the close relation that there is between his neurosis and his whole style of life; the neurosis imposes itself upon him as an illness to be nursed, a disablement that others ought to respect. Wexberg affirms nevertheless that the personality includes and comprehends the neurotic symptom and is responsible for it. That is a directive of cardinal importance in the treatment of the neuroses.

Since it signifies a stoppage or even a retreat before the demands of life, neurosis prevents the individual from accomplishing the three great and fundamental life-tasks which we have already defined. It brings in its train, as a natural consequence, a fear of life which now appears divested of its true significance, and an anguish like that of death.

In the Adlerian view, what matters most is not to discern the form taken by the neurosis but to understand its mechanism. Whereas the causal explanation toils on to a standstill in the multiplicity of the symptoms, the finalist interpretation alone enables us to seize the essential motive. Consider, for example, the case of a man who wants at any cost to avoid conjugal life. From a finalist point of view, the reasons

[1] *International Zeitschrift für Ind. Psychologie*, 3. 1933.

he adduces in explanation of his conduct are obviously not essential, whether he shows himself as impotent, or suffering from a tic, or suddenly finds himself incapable of any activity; since all or any of these symptoms serve the same end —they put marriage out of the question.

The neuroses of children

Bad habits in children are not yet neuroses; we must however recognize that to distinguish between the two is not always easy. The bad habits indicate in any case that the child finds itself in a situation holding some menace to the feeling that it has of its personality, although the nature of the symptom itself is determined by its physical condition. A child with some weakness of the urinary system will wet its bed; another, suffering from a defect of the alimentary canal will have bouts of sickness, etc. What is important from the finalist standpoint is that by this or that means the child wishes to attract the attention of its parents. The notable fact that it produces the troublesome symptom whenever it finds itself in a situation that it feels to be difficult or dangerous is a further proof of the leading rôle played by finality in the neurosis.

The neuroses of adults

It is always the final aim of the personality that precipitates the neurosis, although it is the physical state which conditions the choice of the organ that is to become the seat of nervous disorder. Of all the possible forms of neurosis we will limit ourselves here to the obsessional, which closely resembles the neurosis of anguish.[1] It frequently occurs in individuals who have been pedantically

---

[1] *The neurosis of anguish* is a Freudian term. 'This neurosis . . . defined purely symptomatically, is characterized by its two chief manifestations: the paroxysm of anxiety and a state of chronic anxiety.' R. Dalbiez, *La Methode Psychanalytique*, Vol. 1, p. 388. (Trans.)

brought up, preoccupied since their earliest days, in whatever they may have undertaken, with the idea of attaining absolute perfection. This idea being of course illusory, such persons are never satisfied with what they do, and in everything they do they imitate, though for a very different reason, Penelope at her loom. Their sphere of operation thus becoming narrower and narrower, all fruitful activity at last seems impossible to them, and these unhappy people promptly take cover at the approach of any duty. Yet it is no uncommon thing to hear the people around them complain bitterly about their tyrannical and arrogant behaviour.

To sum up—neurotics are persons who have not managed to compensate their feelings of inferiority in a way that is useful to the community, but have taken a by-path towards some fictive superiority. In order to justify their flight from the obligations that life lays upon all of us, they produce nervous symptoms whose function is to excuse them in their own eyes and those of others. As to the symptoms themselves, they are selected as we have seen, according to the given organic inferiorities.

3. Crime

Like the attitude of the neurotic, but more so, that of the criminal is hostile to society. By what criterion is the one differentiated from the other? First of all by that of the means adopted. The criminal knows that he is behaving as an enemy to society, whilst the neurotic is not aware that his attitude is a-social and does not think that he is responsible. The criminal is more aggressive than the neurotic, because he decides straightway for 'action', and in this he is the nearer to reality. Moreover, the moral consciousness of the criminal is under-developed and his social inhibitions almost non-existent. Is he then courageous? Adler's reply to this surprises some people. Contrary to common opinion, he regards the criminal as a discouraged individual. For him, courage is a quality of the communal feeling, which implies also a settled will to fulfil one's obligations.

In a mortal combat, the weaker may use treachery in order to win despite his inferiority, and this is, at bottom, the fictive 'courage' of the criminal. Genuine courage is that which inspires an objective mode of action—that is, action directed to an end valued for its own sake and not in order to increase the actor's feeling of personality. Nor is it action with a view to the approbation of others, but for the benefit of the community. It is true that we all have need of social approbation, but that is not the prime motive of social action. In default of this approbation, however, the criminal aspires to play a part that will make everyone talk about him, and resorts to antisocial behaviour. Like the neurotic, he wants everyone to recognize his value, but without himself making any positive contribution to the purpose. In the case of the criminal, it may appear that the expense of energy is often excessive for the end in view. But in reality what matters most to him is to prove to himself that he has the 'courage' to live in open revolt against society, and the main-spring of his action will always be the desire for superiority, in whatever guise he strives to attain it.

It is therefore much to be desired that lawyers and magistrates should be psychological as well as casuistical interpreters of the law; for the higher duty of the criminologist should be to understand the personality of the criminal, to explain his error to him and lend a helping hand towards his re-education. The *lex talionis* which even to-day reigns in modified forms, needs to be replaced by a more human law, designed for the restoration to social living of those who have turned against it. That is what would very often happen, if we took the trouble to search out all the influences of which they have been the victims. Every one of us has a share of responsibility for the delinquencies of the criminals, and we ought to do all we can towards their reclamation. The present penal law tends in a quite different direction, in spite of the reformative tendencies making themselves felt here and there. But without waiting for the progress of legal reform, every educator should apply his best efforts to prevent any individual in his care from deviating in the criminal direction. A mature adviser who acts at the same time as a friend, may exert a decisive influence upon a young delinquent; as we shall see later (Chapter Four) in discussing the work of medico-pedagogic councils.

4. *The psychoses*

Not wishing to trespass upon the domain of medicine, we shall say little about the psychoses. The educator need only have sufficient knowledge of this subject not to hesitate about those cases which he will have to refer to the doctor. The great difference between the psychotic and the neurotic is that the former is no longer aware that he is ill; he is living, so to speak, altogether outside reality. The neurotic, on the other hand, is capable of accounting to himself for his condition, and is usually distressed by it. He is able to criticize himself, in which he is unlike the psychotic whose thinking no longer obeys the rules of 'common' sense but those of a purely individual logic. In most psychotic cases a physical inferiority is linked to a cerebral anomaly which no longer permits the normal play of his mental faculties.

The essential point for an educator, is to know at what moment the psychosis in question first appeared, for in almost every case this was during a psychic event which the individual did not know how to cope with.

F. TWO FUNCTIONS OF ADLERIAN PSYCHOLOGY

Adlerian psychology propounds, on the one hand, a *therapy* for the re-education of those persons in whom a feeling of inferiority, reinforced by unfavourable surrounding circumstances, has led into mistaken ways, whether they are ways of neurosis or of delinquency. It proposes, on the other hand, a *prophylaxis*, a preventive and tonic education for the rising generations.

1. *The therapeutic function*

To re-educate a child it is necessary to work at the same time upon its environment, especially upon its parents. The medico-pedagogic councils exist for this purpose; and their task is arduous since the majority of parents are rebellious from the start towards any prescriptions relative to their own conduct. There is need of tact and perseverance, for a series of frequent consultations with the child and with the parents is required if one is to bring about any decisive improvement.

In the treatment of an adult the indispensable condition is the same as it is with children; one has to win the patient's complete confidence. One must apply all one's skill, at first, simply to the understanding of what he says, the interpretation being deferred as secondary. To this end the psychologist allows the patient to express himself with entire freedom, and it is only when the latter seems to have no more to say that he will intervene with a question. In the second phase of the treatment, he will try to show the patient what is mistaken in his behaviour, and the attitude of the patient will become modified in so far as he understands. At a certain moment, a definite relation will establish itself between him and his re-educator. This is the phenomenon to which Freud has given the name of *transference*. The

D   33

patient then becomes aggressive towards the re-educator, whom he will try hard to persuade that his ideas and attitude are wrong and that his method is worthless. It is now of great importance that the practitioner should make the minimum of mistakes, knowing how powerful an influence he can exert by setting the example of a logical attitude in vital crises. In the process of the cure, one should not offer to dispel the symptoms but, above all, completely to alter the patient's attitude to life; for it is then only that he will find the courage to look his duties in the face after having so long evaded them by subterfuges and with innumerable excuses. The therapist ought not to show any personal interest in the patient's recovery, for that would only make it easy for the latter to 'punish' him by taking a still tighter grip of his malady. The patient has to recognize that it is in his own vital interest to be cured, that he must will to be cured, and that he must himself be ready to bear the responsibility of the success or failure of the treatment he has undertaken; for only the individual who can assume a responsibility is on the road to a genuine cure. Beyond this point, Adlerian re-education has the further aim of teaching the individual how to treat himself in the future, so that he will be capable of tackling the many difficulties with which life will not fail to beset his way.

2. *The preventive function*

An education based upon these principles ought as far as possible to leave the child to develop naturally, and to intervene only when necessary. It will endeavour to act upon the child by good example, while doing its best to improve the surrounding familial and social conditions. The constant preoccupation will be to fortify the child's feeling for the community, thereby to develop its confidence in its own capacities, and to help it to compensate its feeling of inferiority, to the utmost possible extent, by courageous activity. For Adler, we must remember, to *educate* is to *encourage*. That is why the educator has always to maintain a benevolent attitude towards the child, showing comradeship towards it under any circumstances, and must never permit this benevolence to be conditional upon the child's performance or behaviour. He should always take the child seriously. Nothing undermines its confidence more than the feeling of not being taken seriously. And there should be no lying to children! This is both useless and dangerous. They have always a right to the truth, though it should be formulated in a manner suitable to their age.

Nor is it a good thing to show anxiety about a child, for such an attitude weakens the self-confidence that it needs to develop: on the contrary, it should be allowed as far as possible to gain experience in its own way. This will always be more profitable to it than the most well-intentioned advice. It is by experiencing the consequences of its own actions that a child learns most quickly to take responsibility for them, and that is the capacity which will be of primary importance to it in all circumstances, at school, at home, and in relations with its play-fellows. Everywhere and always it needs to feel responsibility for what it does. That is the condition *sine qua non* of any full and well-balanced living.

We cannot attempt here to enumerate all the means available to a pedagogy which seeks to proceed upon the principles of Adlerian psychology; we can only indicate a few among the many that present themselves for consideration. The choice of means will obviously depend upon the nature and the surrounding conditions of the child in question.

With children who have a strongly marked tendency to contradict, for example, the wise way is to indicate what they ought to do in the guise of friendly suggestion. If they are little ones, and on the point of doing something silly, it is better to divert their attention than to scold them. Should one ignore a piece of naughtiness in a child? If so, it must be in such a manner that the child does not think it is intentionally overlooked. To copy the child's behaviour in such and such circumstances is a method that is occasionally useful; but it must be used with much circumspection, for irony is a dangerous weapon in pedagogy. Wrongly applied, it can destroy a child's confidence. In some cases, the educator may usefully register extreme astonishment at the pupil's behaviour and show by his attitude that it was the last thing he would have expected of him. However, according to the degree of development a child has attained, one can profitably appeal to its maturity and understanding. Sometimes a gentle imputation of blame is sufficient, and one must know how to avoid actual punishment as far as possible. Above all, and however grave a fault a child may have committed, the educator ought never to deny a child his goodwill. For many children, this benevolence is all too likely to be the one comfort upon which they can rely in a painful, colourless or even miserable life.

G. SUMMARY OF CHAPTER ONE

Adlerian psychology is concerned with the totality of human personality, in which it first distinguishes the different factors and then combines them in their final unity. Its preoccupation is to grasp the whole that the individual constitutes, on the one hand as an independent unity, and on the other hand in its relations with society, since it is only in taking account of the latter that the human being finds its position in its natural environment.

We are thus dealing with a genuine *psychology*, the aim of

which is to understand the human being as concretely as possible.

But this psychology is not directed only towards theoretical knowledge: it offers to provide a basis for a *pedagogy*, a method of education for children and of re-education for adults. These are its preventive and re-educative functions. Is Adlerian psychology a system of ethics? At first sight one is tempted to answer in the affirmative, since it has often to do with values. (The value it accords, for example, to the feeling for community.) However, this would require an attempt to elucidate a point upon which Adlerian psychologists themselves are not too clear. Ethics —one must first define the term—takes us into a realm of norms, of laws and of regulative ideas; it prescribes what must be done to attain to an ideal. One may say, therefore, that an ethics is a system of rules and prescriptions that should regulate our conduct in the name of a higher principle, and that provides us with a scale of values enabling us to judge, in the light of this principle, what is good and what is bad.

Adlerian psychology, however, furnishes no rules, and therefore cannot be conceived as ethics. On the other hand it is related to ethics, because its subject is man in his totality, and man is a moral being. It does, indeed, take man to be naturally good. Its *feeling for community* is a reality pre-existing within us: the task is only to develop it. Dr. Adler insists much upon the moral nature of man without which he could never become a social being. Although, then, we cannot say that Adlerian psychology is ethics in the proper sense of the term, its subject is the individual conceived as a moral being (man is man only in so far as he is moral) and it could be defined as the *science of moral man* (Krauss: *Int. Zeitschr. für Ip.* 4. 1931). And the more so, since it requires of its adherent an unconditional self-dedication.

CHAPTER TWO

Pre-School Education
(*Kindergarten*)

A. FROM BIRTH TO THE AGE OF THREE

KINDERGARTEN is an extension of the education in the family. Let us then begin with a few words about this education within the family during the first years of a child's life when the influence of the mother is of paramount importance. For her, the birth of the infant signifies much more than the mere bodily separation. From the first day of its life the infant constitutes a distinct organism, subject to a finality proper to itself. The maternal duty is, therefore, to assist it in the attainment of a progressively fuller independence; which means that she is no longer to think of the relation between herself and her child as an end in itself. That relation is henceforth only a means towards enabling the child to acquire confidence in itself and the surrounding world; it is the first stage on its way to full membership of the human community.

Small and weak as it is, the infant would perish without someone to take constant care of it. If it is born into a circle insufficiently conscious of this duty towards it, or made up of over-egocentric persons, it will develop the feeling of inferiority to excess. For this reason the mother needs to train herself to think of her child in relation with the world around it and not, as she too often does, only in relation with herself. If she herself exhibits benevolence towards other people, she will develop in the child a similar attitude towards others, and call forth the first signs of that feeling of community which it has to acquire.

We know, indeed, that upon the degree of social confidence that a child possesses depends also its courage, and upon this courage depends its capacity to live—the amount of 'pluck' it will be able to show later, from the very first steps it has to take outside the family circle—in the kindergarten, then in school, and in later life. A good beginning saves it from many subsequent pitfalls, and in any case ensures it against the need, at some future time, of a fundamental re-education.

The attitude assumed by adults towards the child should not be determined by its wishes, but by their concern to facilitate its adaptation to the community. The educator, of all people, cannot afford to take short views, and an immediate objective should never tempt him to forget the final aim, which is always to develop the child's aptitude for co-operation. To take but one example, it is not uncommon for conflicts to arise between small children. Instead of intervening every time, which will accustom them to appeal to adults as the easiest means of self-protection, it is better to leave them to settle the matter by themselves. They will then learn by direct experience that a certain mutual respect is obligatory between equals, and that a state of harmony is better and much more agreeable than one of continual bickering.

We must repeat that children should always be told the truth, with the proviso that it should be given in a form accessible to their understanding. Mendacity on the part of the parents nearly always produces most objectionable consequences, for when one day the child finds out the truth of the matter, it is in danger of losing all filial confidence. That is a serious eventuality, for to a child such a loss of confidence often means the disintegration of its entire world.

There is, for instance, one grave question that children

never fail to raise sooner or later—that of their origin. There is no real reason for not answering this question as calmly and veraciously as any other. If a mother is in expectation of giving the child a brother or sister, this is an excellent way of preparing it for the event, meanwhile giving it to understand that it will soon be the 'bigger one' who will be able to help mother in looking after a little one who will be weak and need so much care, etc. A prudent preparation of this kind from the mother will often, in such a case, protect a child from painful feelings of jealousy and resentment.

B. THE CHILD AT KINDERGARTEN

According to Adler, the kindergarten is the supplementary hand of the family. It ought to carry on what has been well begun; to provide what has been neglected, or to correct what has been done amiss owing to default of understanding or lack of a right environment. But the kindergarten teacher's path bristles with difficulties, for the children brought to her are already little personalities, each with its own directive line of life more or less formed. The kindergarten cannot therefore repair the damages of a bad home-training simply by correcting the child's faults, for whatever were thus eliminated upon the one side would make as troublesome a reappearance on the other. But the kindergarten has to provide a field for such experiences as a mother ought always to permit a child to undergo—namely, those in which confidence can be won. It has to teach the child to think and to act according to 'common' sense, and not according to individual laws (the 'autistic' thinking of Bleuler).

As we have observed, the child's 'style of life' is usually fixed in the course of the first five years, so that the influence exerted by the kindergarten may well be decisive.

All the potentialities of a being are given from its birth. It is a case of developing these: of teaching the child how to avail itself of them. It often happens that capacities that are not at all remarkable in themselves are fulfilled with unexpectedly brilliant results, simply because the appropriate method of training has been found and applied. As we know, the importance of the *attitude* is a kind of *leitmotiv* that runs throughout all Adlerian psychology.

Here is an excessively pampered child, who plays the part of a petty tyrant in his family. From the moment he enters the kindergarten he is continually making scenes. At one time he will disturb his school-mates in the middle of their work, at another time he will plant himself in the centre of attention by steady refusal to do whatever is asked of him. Punishment would serve no purpose: at the best it would make the child apparently more docile, but he would lose little time before producing some other and equally tiresome symptom; such as soiling himself or losing his appetite; and in any case it would worsen his already bad opinion of *other people*. For this child is suffering from being away from his home, where everybody fusses over him and tries to relieve him of every difficulty. The young teacher, therefore, far from punishing such a child will seek to gain its confidence. To this end she will call in the aid of one or more of its playmates, knowing that young children are more readily influenced by one of their own age than by an adult; and as soon as ever the child has learnt to rely upon one—even if no more—of the circle into which it has been transplanted, it will begin to gain the courage of its situation; it will have taken the first step towards communal living.

There are however certain types among children in which the feeling for community cannot develop normally until they have been liberated from a mistaken attitude to life.

Adler distinguishes three of these types:
1. The hated child (gehasstes Kind).
2. The spoilt child (verzärteltes Kind).
3. The child with an organic inferiority (organminder-wertiges Kind).

1. *The hated child*

Like the spoilt child, this type is burdened by too many negative factors to be able to cope with the demands of the community. Never having had the indispensable experience of a mother's understanding, it has never really known what confidence is. Such a child is consequently timid and fearful, and frequently defiant, towards those around it.

2. *The spoilt child*

This type would appear, on the face of things, unlikely to come to such an unfavourable situation as the type which has been denied the love of a mother. Yet it may, for our world has no regard for one who seeks nothing but his own satisfaction. The child who was spoilt at home tries to carry on in the same rôle of the 'unique' one. Disillusion-ment begins, as we have just seen, as soon as he begins to attend kindergarten. Here, since he finds for the first time in his life that he is only one child among all the others, and because they treat him upon the same level as them-selves, he feels as though he had been suddenly plunged into a hostile environment, and, in the effort to subdue it to his caprice, as he could always do at home, he is tempted to resort to the tricks of rebellion. It is now the task of the teacher to get him to abandon these ways and to direct him into those of the community.

3. *The child with an organic inferiority*

In this child the feeling for community is sure to be

deficient. Suffering from an organic condition with which
he is constantly preoccupied, his interest is too much concentrated upon himself, and since every effort is painful to
him he seeks for ways around every obstacle: having little
self-assurance, he is apt to be quickly overcome by discouragement. When one has to deal with a child of this
type one must try to train it with a view to some compensation for its organic inferiority. And if it should in fact *over-
compensate* it may even achieve something above the average.
One will do well, however, to have had it previously examined
by a doctor, in order to make sure that there is not also a
mental defect prejudicial to its normal development.

Particular attention ought to be given to *clumsy* children,
whose awkwardness is often apparent in the difficulty with
which they learn to read and write. For instance the child
who suffers from a weakness of its right hand is easily made
to feel inferior and surrounded, as it were, by enemies. One
should therefore encourage it, partly by giving attention
to any superiority it has in other respects, and partly by
allowing it to use both hands indifferently; which may even
be of advantage to it in later life.

Those who frequent kindergarten schools soon notice
how a child likes to play a certain *rôle*. Dr. Adler emphasizes
the importance of the rôle that a child chooses (Rollenspiel)
for this invariably yields invaluable information about its
personality. For example, a child who always wants to be
the leader, whether the game is about railways or police-
men, shows evident need to command, if only in the realm
of fantasy. He wants, then, to be strong. In collective games,
it is always the same children who want to give the direc-
tions, just as we find it is the same ones who obediently
follow them. The kindergarten will teach the former to
obey at least once (whoever wants to command must first
learn to obey) and will encourage the timid ones to take

initiative, and little by little to free themselves from the tutelage of the authoritarians. On the other hand, the parts that children choose to play can provide useful indications as to the prevailing atmosphere of the domestic fireside (when, for example, a child imitates the father scolding the mother, or wants to throw everything around it down to the floor).

In order to train the senses of these little ones and, at the same time, their capacity to co-operate, one devotes certain periods to individually educative games and others to collective activities, whether of work or play.

4. *Comparison between an Adlerian and a Montessorian kindergarten*

To turn the findings of psychology to the advantage of pedagogy, to complete the family phase of education, prepare the child for school, and to endeavour to bring it to the stage of development normal for a child of six—these are the preoccupations of an Adlerian kindergarten. During such a preparation this kindergarten will, in conformity with Adler's teaching, endeavour above all to render the child independent, able to adapt itself to the new situations which life will be continually presenting to it; and for this the *free method* seems to Adler the best. Since however he is far from wishing to be original at all costs, he is not afraid of recommending what seems to him to be good in the methods of Montessori and Froebel.

Nevertheless, those methods are markedly different. In a Montessorian kindergarten, for instance, the discipline is settled once and for all—involving an enormous initial labour—after which the child has to learn to follow certain rules rather than to develop its own capacity for adaptation. It is a very good thing for the teacher as far as possible to efface herself, as Montessorian teachers do, but then one can hardly prevent much of the authority passing over to the material means employed—means which, we willingly concede, are indeed of immense value for the training of the senses.

What has impressed us as something not quite natural, when we have been visiting Montessorian kindergartens, is that one hears no noises in them. The children work in silence at their little tables; if they have to move from one place to another they go on tip-toe. One never hears them cry or sees them run, and it would seem impossible for two of them to quarrel. Judged from these appearances, the discipline of an Adlerian school is nothing like so good. But the little community that it constitutes, if obviously less orderly, reveals itself to deeper observation as all the more intimate and valuable, since it allows the child to move about in complete freedom as in the bosom of a big family. Moreover it may happen, as it will in a family, that one child will rebel, or want to play with another, or that a boy will amuse himself teasing a little girl. All these little upsets are incidental to daily life, and a kindergarten cannot do better than accustom children to cope with them in common. From its point of view, it is more important to shape these little beings for communal living than to make them read and write before they go to school, where they may feel bored in the midst of more backward schoolfellows. That is why the Adlerian kindergarten attaches such importance to personal creative work, which takes only a secondary place in the Montessorian kindergarten. On the whole, the Montessorian method does little for the communal training of the children, each working alone at its little desk. They only come together in the period of silence, in the intuitive lessons, the rhythmic exercises and some outdoor games. This strikes us as insufficient, in view of the long hours children spend in these kindergartens— from nine in the morning to five or six in the evening.

The development of a communal feeling has moreover a happy influence upon the children's speaking. Many of them, who still express themselves with difficulty when they enter the Adlerian kindergarten, rapidly learn to converse, thanks to the mutual contacts it encourages them to make. One has often been able to verify the fact that a child's vocabulary increases and its speaking improves progressively as it becomes more social. Adler has observed that the children who are most backward in learning to talk—excepting of course those hindered by organic defects—are the spoilt children. They have not hitherto felt much need to speak, since all their desires have been satisfied by those around them, without their having to take much pains to be understood. A poorly developed speech is thus a sign that the child is still egocentric and its communal feeling as yet only feeble.

To sum up; the kindergarten based upon Adlerian principles is in truth a school of life: it forms a little society, of a very natural kind, approximating as nearly as possible to the family, where the child learns to become independent, to collaborate and makes friends, having also time and opportunity to gain individual experience.

By way of example, here is an account of a morning spent in an Adlerian kindergarten—that of Dr. Friedmann:

At half-past eight in the morning the children arrive, each brought by its mother or a nurse. Entering the cloak-room, they take off their outdoor things each by itself. Some are not good at this, but no one gets impatient, there is no hurry; a cleverer schoolfellow simply shows them what they have to do.

Having donned a little brightly-coloured apron, the child then enters the class. Free as it is from any constraint, it is interesting to note how its bearing differs from day to day according to its moods. One day it will make its entry into

46

the class-room at a skip and a run, or puff around it for a minute or more 'like a railway engine'. On another day it is no sooner in the room but it plunges into a game upon which it will spend itself for nearly an hour with extraordinary ardour. Yet another day it will make a sedate entry, leading in a more timid little class-mate.

When the whole class is assembled the children resume the work that was begun on the preceding day, or they decide what they would like to do next. Several children may sit down together at a small table; some cutting out paper shapes while others wield the gum-brush; others again are building with blocks. Each child is allowed to follow its bent, with the sole reservation that it should never begin a new task before finishing what it was doing before.

Just before ten o'clock these proceedings are suspended and a few pupils begin eagerly to lay the main table, which it is a great honour to be asked to do. The plates are arranged and the meal begins. The children have brought this with them, and as they come from very different homes, their provisions also are very unequal. These range from pieces of bread, often pretty dry, to well-buttered slices, fruit and chocolate . . . it is a situation well worth watching.

The little people begin with a silent, intense, ocular comparison between what the others have brought and what they have themselves. Certain mutual presentations ensue, occasionally even complete exchanges. Some of the children offer others a taste of something they think particularly good, but only to their special friends, while others display the same liberality but include the whole company. A few, on the contrary, do not want to share anything at all, though before long they get drawn in by the good examples. The collation having been disposed of, two or three children undertake to clear the table and sweep up the crumbs.

The hour that follows is usually devoted to a little general conversation. The children are, for instance, led to discuss the best ways of taking off their things; or the proper way to behave towards a playfellow in such and such a case; or one may set them some little problem concerning the sharing of provisions, etc.

After this, there is a period of rhythmic exercise. The children enjoy this enormously, all without exception; they find equal satisfaction in it from the most timid to the most obstreperous. For them it is without doubt the finest moment of the whole morning. They then get ready to go to play in the park. This happens to be ten minutes away, and to get there the children have to cross a road filled with heavy traffic; an inconvenience which has its advantage since they begin to learn how to get about with safety, a matter of some importance to life in a great city. Once they are in the park they are at complete liberty and take full advantage of it to play, shout and run about; but they come back promptly to their teacher whenever she calls. For their liberty, far from being a symptom of disorder, has been earned little by little, just so far as they have proved worthy of it.

Such as it is—for an institution that means to follow life, and never to become the slave of its routine, will have constantly to seek improvements—this kindergarten renders genuine services, as much in the assistance of home education as in the preparation of the child for school. For it strengthens and trains in the infant that communal sense which is beyond all price, its capacity for adaptation to circumstances, and its confidence in itself and in others. It is the children with these qualities who will be men and women of the future in the best sense of the words—those who will joyfully fulfil the responsibilities laid upon them by membership of the community of mankind.

CHAPTER THREE

The Adlerian Experimental School
(*Individualpsychologische Versuchsschule*)

WHAT is this experimental school, founded in September 1931, whose existence remained unknown to many school-managers in Vienna itself, even after it had begun to enjoy a well-deserved reputation abroad? At first it appeared to be nothing out of the ordinary. This high school for boys ('Hauptschule' comprises the fifth to the eighth forms) is hardly distinguishable from the other 'Wiener Hauptschulen' which had all, since 1926, undergone a valuable reformation.[1] A superficial visitor could easily fail even to notice the spirit that pervades this establishment. Let us inspect it, then, with our eyes well open.

Poor enough in appearance, the school building is situated in an impoverished quarter of the twentieth district, where a population which could earn only a bare living in normal times is now suffering cruelly from unemployment. The children often arrive at school in lamentable condition. On many occasions, in the depth of winter, we have seen them hungry and shivering with cold. The school itself is very badly warmed, for it lacks the money to procure a sufficiency of fuel—some class-rooms are occupied until six in the evening, yet the heat is turned off from ten in the morning. For this reason the opening of windows in winter time is not allowed during the recreation periods, even though these have to be spent in class for lack of a courtyard or any other open-air playground. These deplorable conditions cannot fail to make their depressing

[1] Cf. Dottrens, *L'éducation nouvelle en Autriche.*

influence felt throughout the schooling of these necessitous children.[1] If such a school, then, manages to give positive results, if it can already claim many successes, they cannot be attributed to external conditions particularly appropriate to children's needs.

The teachers in this experimental school—amongst whom we have previously mentioned Drs. Spiel, Birnbaum and Scharmer with our personal gratitude—merit the recognition due to everyone who devotes himself body and soul to the high calling of education. These are teachers who succeed in creating a purer atmosphere around them, enabling their little pupils to forget the poverty that weighs so heavily on their frail shoulders. It is to them that these children owe the only bright hours of their sombre existence, and in the memory of such great friends they may well find an abiding encouragement. We experienced in ourselves the vivifying effect of their example, that of educators whose work is a vocation in the noblest meaning of the word. The tireless enthusiasm of their work and their skill in gaining the children's confidence make us think of them as artists, and of their magnanimity as that of priests. Such a capacity to make the mind radiate and triumph over circumstance commands our deepest admiration.

And with what inexhaustible patience they had to persevere to be allowed to do this work! Their first success, when they obtained the provisional foundation of an experimental school of Adlerian pedagogy, was the late fruit of more than ten years of preparatory labour. On 15th September, 1931, came the reward of their efforts; the school was approved by the State school authority of Vienna, and they could then proceed to its official establishment. Besides the three teachers we have named, who are still the soul of the institution, masters were appointed who were interested in

[1] Upon this subject, see H. Hetzer, *Kindheit und Armut*.

the new methods and already possessed some competence in them. Thus, before the winning of official approbation, the amount of work that had to be done must not be underrated. United in a spirit of rare collaboration, Drs. Spiel, Birnbaum and Scharmer were at the same time extremely strict with one another. They were present in turn at each other's lessons and were not sparing of mutual criticism. Many times, as they admitted to us, they came to the brink of despair about the whole undertaking: but one or another of them always succeeded in reviving the damaged morale of his colleagues; and each time a new impulse, a fresh access of strength enabled them to attack their problem with yet greater ardour.

To follow the work of such a school from day to day is to realize that there are indeed masters who are 'artists', for whom the Adlerian psychology has become a veritable reason for living, whilst some others remain only practitioners who may have fully adopted the new method, but are still using it, so to speak, from outside, the ideas themselves not having touched or transformed them inwardly. In the latter case the advantage gained by the new ideas is evidently smaller, but it is still real, for the children learn, all the same, how to surmount the obstacles that daily life presents to them in an atmosphere of co-operation and mutual understanding. It must be understood, of course, that this is not to defend an attitude which in itself is defective, but merely to say that the drawback seems in practice less serious than might be expected.

One commonly distinguishes education as an end in itself from the ends that it seeks to attain (the purely scholastic aims), and that not without reason. We shall now see how incomparably well this school manages to reconcile these two aspects of education in a synthesis to which so many teachers have aspired in vain.

THE ADLERIAN EXPERIMENTAL SCHOOL

A. THE AIMS OF INSTRUCTION

These aims are the same as in the other State schools, since one of the conditions laid down at the opening of the experimental school was that they should exactly conform to the ordinary syllabus of the *Hauptschulen* so that any change in this respect was excluded in advance. However, since the 'active school' methods were introduced in nearly all Viennese schools after the great reform of 1926, it is safe to say that there has been a general improvement of instruction. This progress is at once evident in the arrangement of the classes. The desks are no longer ranked one behind another as they used to be, but are disposed in a semi-circle, so that the majority of the pupils see one another's faces. The walls are hung with photographs and engravings cut from the illustrated journals or with drawings made in the class, which have some bearing upon the lessons in geography, or in science (sketches of machines etc.), or natural history (animals and plants), or in mathematics (figures and formulae), or relating to their collective discussions (diagrams recording something to this purpose), etc. In all these schools, too, there are geography rooms with sand relief maps, and scientific laboratories.

In these schools the active method is now employed in the majority of classes, up to the age of twelve or thirteen, with, of course, greater or lesser ingenuity. The putting into practice of the principles of the active school beyond its indicated limits appears to be hardly possible at present. The programmes of the colleges are so overcharged that the teachers are obliged to resort to the old authoritarian methods, the sole object of which is to inculcate the greatest possible quantity of knowledge. This means that freedom in the work and the spirit of true collaboration decline as the pupil rises from class to class, except in the scientific subjects where the co-operative spirit has been proving its value for many years. This too rapid ascent of the instructional ladder prevents any stopping to attend to the laggards: and the pupil whose rhythm is somewhat slow, though he may be as intelligent as his quicker neighbour, is invariably sacrificed. This may be an 'aristocratic' principle, concerned above all to produce an *élite*, but the democratic ideal is to raise the whole mass to as high a level as possible. This fundamental difference, in a matter of principle which pervades the life of every day, does not fail to make itself felt to-day in the little republic, not yet fully able to free itself from age-old ideas.

Though the principles of the active school have been assimilated by the majority of the masters, the practice of them takes on a special aspect in the experimental school based upon Adler's psychology. For it is in this school that the desire of the masters to bring about the progress of all the pupils without distinction is most clearly evident: it is in this school alone that we have seen them attend to each one with an equal devotion. It has most happily profited by the Adlerian discovery that a bad school record is more often due to a child's lack of courage, perhaps caused by its first defeat, than to a lack of aptitude—a discovery to which so many now owe the recovery of their lost confidence.

When he has a new class to teach, the Adlerian teacher quickly estimates the difference between the pupils who are already 'gifted' in whatever direction, and those who are not so yet. And he will then treat the former like 'practised hands', while taking the utmost pains to interest the latter in the subject under consideration. Towards them he will use the 'propaganda technique' of Birnbaum until he has fully awakened the interest that was lacking in them.

As to *punishment*, the part it plays in this school is very different from what one finds elsewhere. For example, it is hardly ever imposed for negligence in the fulfilment of a task. Not that Adlerians expect to abolish all punishments in a day; they expect rather to be able to eliminate them little by little, till in the end they become quite needless. At first blush such an ambition appears perfectly monstrous in the eyes of many educators, but it is a fact that these Viennese masters are getting nearer to its realization every day. The fruitfulness of the Adlerian method is shown above all in its practical effects. In our opinion, those who have not visited this school and inspected the work it is doing ought to abstain from a definitive judgement upon Adlerian psychology; for it is only on consideration of what it has managed to achieve in spite of the worst conditions, that one can render it full justice.

If one compares a lesson given in the Adlerian school with a lesson in an ordinary school (both applying the 'active' system so far as is possible with classes of thirty to forty pupils) one must certainly admit the difference of atmosphere. The experimental school is in advance of the others. In theory their objectives are the same; both are trying to train their pupils in independence and in aptitude for co-operation. But the way that the means to this are used are from the first divergent, and the results obtained have very little in common. In many classes of the other schools, teachers who are overburdened and overstrained content themselves with the pursuit of ends that are, so to speak, external. By their own account—though there are certainly exceptions—they can do no more, and to go beyond a formal training (Adler and Birnbaum's 'äusseres Training') seems to them Utopian. This training would doubtless amount to a good deal, if in later life the pupils really became capable of using it to full advantage. But the object of the active schools is still the acquisition of the largest possible quantity of information; and the question is whether the means employed to achieve this are the most reasonable and appropriate to the child's development. The assimilation of so many subjects exacts the best exertions both of the teacher and of the pupils, so that the educational aim becomes a secondary consideration—even consciously so to a number of teachers, whose attitude is partly excusable in view of the frightful mass of information that is nowadays expected of applicants for the most modest situations. The terrible unemployment crisis, when there was so little demand for labour, had the all too natural effect of causing the employers to raise the standards of qualification.

It is moreover a deplorable fact, which we mention in passing, and one that could be verified in any large town, that of those workers who are regarded as privileged because they have work, many are literally exhausted by the effort it demands. The exertions they have to put forth to make both ends meet are such that their lot is not after all much better than that of the unemployed.

These considerations are all relevant, if we are to understand how commonly both master and pupil are haunted by the question of employment, and why they stake all their hopes of solving it upon taking the greatest range of subjects. A good all-round character is not enough, in these days, to make up for lack of exact knowledge in a given situation. The standard schooling therefore tries to teach as many subjects as it can, so that its pupils may be able, later on, to show some knowledge of any occupation in which a vacant situation may present itself. The choice of a career in advance has become little more than a dream!

What, then, can the experimental school do to improve its teaching, confronted as it is by the same conditions as are the ordinary schools? Thanks to the exceptional qualities of its masters, it manages to supplement its teaching by a genuine *interior* training. In the course of his daily instruction, the master seeks to know each pupil as an individual, and help him to discover his own best ways of working and learning.

But before proceeding to the educational aim, we must glance at the question of examinations, which recur twice every year (15th February and 15th July). A custom peculiar to Vienna is to distribute certificates twice annually, dividing the school year into two five-monthly periods. At the end of each period the newspapers regularly contain articles about the suicides of scholars, with exhortations to parents not to attach over-importance to school reports, not to strike children, nor to threaten them with excessive punishments, etc. This agonizing experience recurs twice yearly, in spite of all that the psychologists and educators of Vienna have so far tried in order to improve the lot of the scholars. Dr. Spiel, the great teacher of the experimental school, delivered a lecture on this subject nineteen times in two weeks before parents' meetings, in most of the districts of Vienna. He explained to these parents the value formerly set upon these reports and what importance one should now attribute to them. In the old school, examiners depended essentially on what had been learnt by heart and whoever had the best memory was considered the best pupil. In our days it is different; we want our students above all to learn to reason correctly and to make the best possible use of all their faculties. To discern and estimate the child's memory is not enough for the modern teacher, who takes just as much interest in the development of the infant's reasoning, in the imagination of his pupils, in their rhythm of work and of assimilation (Arbeitstempo).

He strives moreover to know their characters, and their intimate behaviour. School reports record only specific performances, and parents should never forget that they imply no general judgement on a pupil. One need only analyse the procedure by which reports are made to see how very relative they are.

The teacher may first of all proceed by comparison, estimating his pupils' performances relatively. He may also take account of the child's environment, reckoning, for instance, that a child brought up in a bourgeois home should write a composition more easily than a working-class child, having presumably a richer vocabulary. This done, he compares the child's performance with what he thinks should be expected, considering its capacities. The master may, however, simply take the syllabus as his basis, and evaluate the pupils' exercises according to what is considered normal in the same class. Nor should parents forget that the reports also depend partly upon the master's personality however conscientious he may be. He remains only a man, and we know that each man has his own view of life, his special conception of the world, personal convictions which inevitably sway his judgement. Thus, one master may naturally prefer work that is dryly objective while another responds readily to what is individual. An average pupil, changing to another school, may find himself suddenly in an unusually good class in which he has to take a low place: but the same pupil, if transferred to a weaker class, would have risen to the top of it. After all, said Dr. Spiel to these parents, reports are really important only to the educator and to the child: they speak as it were a private language, the one saying to the other 'This is where you are, and that is where you want to be.'

Any final verdict upon a child needs to be based upon both a pedagogic judgement and a psychological judgement. Here, for example, is a child who succeeds very well in every subject but arithmetic, in which it fails regularly.

Upon inquiry we learn that its father is particularly good at figures, and keen to see his boy become an accountant. At first everything goes well with him at school. But then our little accountant-to-be is presented with a baby sister, to whom the father pays so much tender attention that he rather neglects his first-born. One fine day, the boy runs to his father for help in answering an arithmetical question, upon which the latter puts the little girl aside and gives the most generous attention to his son's inquiry. In that moment the child has unconsciously acquired an experience which will enable him always to attract his father's attention. Is it any wonder that he begins to go from bad to worse in arithmetic till he is nearly at the bottom of the class? For we now know that he has 'need' of this means, to convince himself of his father's affection, of which, rightly or wrongly, he had felt himself frustrated since the birth of his sister. Confronted with a case of this kind the teacher's duty is, first, to unravel the tangle of factors involved, and then simply to explain them in terms the child can understand. Then, without the child's noticing it, he will begin again by setting it a problem a little easier than usual, in solving which it may regain reliance upon its own ability. And after some gradual retraining, little by little, in harder problems this child will recover its position as one of the best pupils in arithmetic, to which it was entitled by its intelligence.

If parents took account of all the factors influencing the allocation of marks, they would be unlikely to attach such importance to them. They should try to realize clearly how difficult it is for a conscientious master to classify children by awarding marks. But the co-operation of both parents and teachers will be needed to prevent the excessive anxiety that many children feel at the approach of the examinations.

B. THE EDUCATIVE AIM

Far from ascribing exaggerated importance to knowledge, Adlerian psychology tends to subordinate instruction to the integral aim of education; that is, as far as possible, for it remains always necessary to fulfil the regular syllabus of the public schools.

For this psychology, the essential aim is the right development of all the faculties, the formation of personalities, free but capable of co-operation, and the awakening in the children of the will to surpass themselves. It seeks to give each one the means of continuing its self-education in later life: and a teacher who has guided his pupil to the point at which the latter is capable of carrying on by himself may consider his task accomplished. All genuine education ought to lead on to this self-education, which is the *sine qua non* of progress in the true sense of the word. Thus alone can the children of to-day become the men of to-morrow. The Adlerian school, then, avoids giving excessive importance to the immediate object of most of the schools, which are content simply to put the pupil in a position to earn his keep at school-leaving age. It looks beyond this, affirming in hope and faith the eternal human values, and strives to overcome the troubles of our times by the formation of men of character. And for all their material worries, the children here do learn what are the great problems of mankind and how true values are to be found. Much that religion was formerly thought to give is to be found here, permeating every lesson. Where the family, disintegrated as it is by disastrous historical circumstances, cannot supply the respect and admiration which are the foundations of all religious feeling (Bovet), it devolves upon the school to supply this grave deficiency. The experimental school-founders knew this. The example set by its teachers would be sufficient to awaken these sentiments in the children. But they also do more and better than that.

The active school method serves only as the basis of their work. There are two things the children have to learn: on the one hand to enter into full contact with the class, the parents and the teachers; and on the other hand to become as independent as they can. These requirements may at first look contradictory, but experience proves that it is only to the degree that a person attains independence that he becomes capable of real co-operation.

In the experimental school, both activity and learning are ruled by the idea of *community* (Gemeinschaft). The group brought together by circumstances into the same class-room furnishes but a case in point. For this group is far from being a real community, which it can become only at the end of a long and persevering endeavour. Indeed, this group begins as a mere collocation of units, without any internal cohesion, whereas the community it is to become should be a new entity, capable of putting forth efforts far superior to those of any isolated individual. The task is the heavier because no prior selection has been possible, such as might have made this transformation easier. While directing the forces at his disposal and developing those that are only latent, the teacher will try to find a place for every individual, to help each one to become of some use to all. He will awaken those tendencies that appear to him desirable, and perhaps canalize others that are opposed or dangerous to the community. What means ought he to employ to this end? Few words and many deeds. For an experience gained in community is of more efficacy than many long and unexceptionable lectures. All the exertions of an Adlerian master are directed to the same end—the creation of a community sense, that will link together, by innumerable unseen ties, these thirty or forty human beings who are thrown together and who have now to meet and surmount their difficulties in common, to share their setbacks and their satisfactions. Only in that way can a condition that in itself is more or less insupportable become an inexhaustible source of strength for all. For Adler, as we saw, perfect community is an ideal never wholly realized by any community whatever. He regards it as a transcendent aim to which one can but progressively approach; and of school communities the best is only partly successful. It takes on different forms according to circumstances.

1. *The work-community* (Arbeitsgemeinschaft)

This is the least characteristic feature of the experimental school, for we found it equally well realized in most other Viennese schools. It proceeds on the active principle, most intelligently adapted to the requirements of large public schools. The master tries to make himself—so far as the crowded curriculum allows—the *primus inter pares*. He encourages original and personal work as much as he can, allowing the children to seek and find for themselves what used to be presented to them 'pre-masticated'. This aim is pursued, we must repeat, within limits restricted by necessity. But what a pleasure it was to see a whole class in eager and animated discussion upon a question raised by one of the pupils—for example, why has Sweden so warm a climate while Greenland has a polar climate, both at the same latitude? It was about half an hour before one of them thought of mentioning the Gulf Stream. Then, and not till then, the master took the floor to complete and correct the explanation that the pupils themselves had put forward. We are very sure that not one of these children will in future forget the capital importance of this factor in the European climate.

To consider, for the moment, only the character of the

'lessons' themselves, we were struck by one practice that seemed to be general in the public schools: the lessons in, e.g., geography given by the same master to different classes were all extraordinarily similar. We were tempted to say too much so, and we often found it hard to resist an impression that the teachers had adopted a new technique of instruction (the active school) once and for all; that they had set up new but definitive limitations and new rules, more spacious certainly than those of old but apparently just as unalterable. There are many points at which routine, that worst enemy of life and progress, is already beginning to exert its ossifying influence. One symptom is that the masters behave as if they knew beforehand just how a lesson will proceed, and fix in advance how much time they will allot to this or that question. The pupils have to put up their hands for the right to speak—a bad old practice that few teachers know how to dispense with—and this cannot but impose a certain passivity upon the pupils. They do avail themselves of a trifle more freedom than before, but it amounts to little more than a less rigid regard for the rules of yesterday. It is far from constituting a positive factor, acquired by the children after a long series of efforts and therefore deserved by them. It is of course true that many people think of freedom as a mere absence of rules, but reason is on the side of those who regard it as that degree of autonomy which an individual is able to attain. Most teachers of the active school have but imperfectly grasped the right conception of freedom: those who know how to avoid these mistakes are exceptions.

The Adlerian experimental school, however, is not content with the arousing of the pupils' spontaneous activity, nor does it limit itself to creating community in learning. It goes further; we would even venture to say that its essential aim begins where the work of most of the other schools finishes. In this school we have had the enjoyable and unforgettable privilege of taking part in an education that is firmly wedded to life. And here two lessons are never the same, although given by the same master upon the same subject.

Here is the true realization of the active method, a school continually adapted to the interests and requirements of its pupils!

2. *The administrative community* (Verwaltungsgemeinschaft)

This communal activity is established in most of the schools, but as we shall see it acquires a particular aspect in the case of the Adlerian school. In the ordinary schools there are many classes that have successfully achieved 'self-government', but experience has shown that the great majority of teachers do not altogether approve of it. More often than not it stops half-way, for lack of motive power. Must we lay the blame to the excess of work? However that may be, the prefects and monitors too often behave like officials acting upon authority borrowed from the masters, to whom, moreover, they do not hesitate to refer in many cases. At bottom, it is no very great advance from schools that apply the 'firm method' (which relies on the teachers to pronounce judgement with authority and impartiality) to those in which a group of the pupils reward and punish their comrades. The judges are not the same, but we are still just as far from the Adlerian ideal of rendering all punishment superfluous. What matters to the Adlerian is that the child should learn to develop its personality and remain true to it while respecting that of its comrades. Such an education is not easy, but it will be invaluable to a pupil all his life, whatever career he may embrace. And if he is to acquire knowledge and control of himself, he must understand the deeper reasons for the successes as well

as for the set-backs of his earlier life, for with this knowledge alone can he go on to his self-education. It is only by
governing themselves that children gain the perspicacity
to distinguish the situations in which they can 'give a lead'
from those in which their duty is to submit to the community. Taking more pains to understand the actions of the
others than to judge them, they will then make the effort
needed to put themselves in the place of this or that schoolfellow, and will explain to him any mistake he may have
made, showing him also how he ought to behave in any
similar case in the future. A child thus admonished feels
relieved, as it were, of a burden that had oppressed it;
and in recognizing its error it feels, perhaps for the first
time, what it is to be responsible.

Order is entirely administered by the pupils. There are
a first and a second head pupil, and the whole class is
divided into groups of from five to seven pupils, each with
its own leader. The latter renders to the head of the class
an account of the work and behaviour of his group-members at the end of each week.

3. *The community of conversation* (Aussprachegemeinschaft)

This is closely linked to the administrative community.
There is a fixed period each week for general conversation
(Klassenbesprechungen) in which the children discuss what
they have been doing. Here we have a practice characteristic of the Adlerian school. Of the sixty classes in other
public schools that we visited, we found only one that
practised this discussion in common; and upon making
closer acquaintance with the teacher in charge we discovered that she was a fervent disciple of Dr. Adler. This
was Fräulein Régine Seidler, to whom we owe particular
gratitude for the unforgettable lessons she allowed us to
witness. We shall refer to them again later.

It is no light task to draw children of ten into general conversation. The central problem is that of *discipline*. The children have to learn to listen to the one who is speaking, to control themselves and not to speak all at once. They have to learn to reflect upon the qualities required of a head pupil, and of the other members of the class. The masters have had to acquire their own experience in this business. When they began by allowing too much liberty it very soon degenerated into anarchy, and they were obliged to take the reins more firmly into their own hands. They could relax them again only little by little, just to the degree that the class improved in self-control. One is made immediately aware of the 'acquired' character of any freedom that is to be genuine 'self-government'.

The *individual conversations* (Einzelbesprechungen) carried on at the same time as the general discussions, again revealed the devotion of these teachers (who sacrifice much of their own time to their pupils outside school hours). Always at the disposal of anyone who has the desire or the need to confide in him, the Adlerian schoolmaster never hesitates to call to his side a pupil with whom he thinks he has not yet made sufficient contact. The two kinds of conversation complement one another, with the happiest consequences for the class as a whole.

The master is never content with being a good observer. He may notice, for instance, some malicious traits in a certain child. Punishment would very likely estrange the child from him, and even if punishment made it behave better there would probably be no genuine change. For the child's directive 'line of life' would not be modified, and upon finding itself again in similar circumstances it would fall back upon the same conduct as before, that of an enemy to the community. In Adlerian psychology it is the duty of the teacher to discover the life-style of such a child, and to assist it in the construction of a new one that will enable it to develop in harmony with its fellows. We have seen that the disappearance of tiresome symptoms signifies nothing of itself; that one has to penetrate the unconscious of a child in order to uncover the aim that it so obstinately wants to pursue by means hostile to the community. A child that has but once recognized the error in its conduct is already not the same, and that is the moment when re-education can begin. Something must break down before one can reconstruct.

In certain cases the master will not hesitate to resort to slight subterfuges that may influence the child beneficially. Knowing, for example, that one of his boys, at present in a phase of discouragement, has read a book that the others are unlikely to know, he may steer the conversation towards a subject which enables him to ask, as though by the way—'Have any of you happened to read that book?' The eyes of the boy in question at once confirm what was already known to the master, who, by inviting him to speak, puts him in a position of advantage. Little artifices like this can work wonders.

Finally, the master acts as a *trainer*, by knowing how to keep the right way between two indispensable aims—those of encouraging the child and of diminishing its egocentricity (Abbau der Ichhaftigkeit). In the training of each pupil the educator needs to take account of all the given factors—the state of its health, its behaviour in class, the influences from its family, the neighbourhood it comes from, and the company it keeps.

This is to say that the educator is in need of the *regular assistance of the parents*, which is perhaps of all things the hardest to obtain. But in spite of its ever-renewed difficulty, this is a point upon which the Adlerian school has never given in. Each master appoints certain hours at which he is at the parents' disposition. The interviews demand great delicacy, for the teacher needs to learn all kinds of things about the child, but must never make the father or mother feel he is inquisitive: such a feeling would finally alienate them from the school. He has to convince them that their collaboration aids him in his work, and must never lead them to believe that it is the child's ill-behaviour that has obliged him to make contact with them. In many parents one finds traces of this prejudice, that there is something disgraceful about being called in by the teacher. However, at Vienna there are monthly parents' reunions (Eltern-vereinigungen), open to all parents of pupils of the same school, and the recorded attendance is of 50–70 per cent, from which one may infer that the interest of parents in educational questions is growing. Here they have oppor-tunities of hearing addresses by experienced teachers upon subjects of immediate interest to them. While thus pro-viding matter for reflection, the speakers teach them how to supervise their children's behaviour and to some extent their own as well. Little by little, a much-needed education in parenthood is beginning. Whenever some subject happens to arouse special interest in one of the classes, the master invites all his pupils one evening for a perfectly frank talk with them: and it is a most moving experience to see a simple workman, when such a discussion has turned his attention inward upon himself, and revealed things he had never before suspected, awakening to a wholly new interest in life. At the break-up of one of these meetings we have overheard such comments as these:

'If they had only told us that in *our* school days!'

'If only we'd known that a child's mind is like that!'

In a few districts, where the reception of this teaching is especially rewarding, classes are arranged for par-ental advice (Elternratschule). Here parents are initiated by, for example, a series of eight lectures in the basic principles of Adlerian psychology. The medico-pedagogic councils, of which we shall speak in the next chapter, contribute equally to the education of the parents.

If this education is the hardest of all tasks, it is also the one that yields the richest results, collaboration between parent and teacher being indispensable to full educational success. Without it, the best efforts fall short of their aim. One must always try to win the parents' confidence and interest them more and more in the fulfilment of this paramount duty to posterity. The closer the collaboration, the less need there will be for punishments, until at last they will be superseded. Then we may adopt Nietzsche's opinion —'The day is dawning when we shall perhaps know nothing else but education.'

4. *The community of mutual aid* (Stützungsgemeinschaft)

This comprises every exercise of the most immediate duty incumbent upon a community. For example, the child who is good at reading is seated next to another who is weak in that respect. *Per contra*, the one whose reading is poor may be good at arithmetic; it is incumbent on him, in turn, to help a neighbour who is weaker at it; and so on in every subject. One tries, whenever possible, to put a good pupil near a backward one, so that he may learn to understand his comrade's difficulties and help him with them. Friends in need are rare, according to an old proverb, but we can bear witness that this is definitely contradicted by the behaviour of these children. They are a living community, they reckon quite as much with their comrades' needs as their own, and are as concerned about the set-backs of their friends as about their own mistakes. Such a community illustrates the greatness of the idea 'Each for all and all for each'. These children are commencing, in class and under the guidance of a great friend, that apprenticeship to life which they will have to complete later under inevitably harsh conditions.

We must here refer to a characteristic of all the Viennese schools: the bisection of each class into sections A and B.

The former are of those who learn more quickly. Their syllabus includes more than that of the same Class B, whose rhythm of work is slower. Pupils in A classes have the right to pass later into the secondary schools and colleges (Mittelschulen) whilst a pupil of Class B, after having completed the four classes of the High School, has no right of entry into another school. The distinction is arrived at as follows: the teacher at the primary school (Volksschule), who has followed his pupil's progress for four years, fills in a form upon his aptitudes (Schülerbeschreibungsbogen). This form accompanies the pupil to the school to which he is transferred. The form is made out upon the basis of a highly-detailed questionary, for upon it will depend the position of the child in the High School from the fifth to the eighth year of his schooling. We must add, however, that the masters of these classes have the right, at a later date, to promote a promising pupil of category B to category A, or *vice versa* for a pupil who turns out to be duller than had been supposed.

Such changes, however, are rarely necessary, which shows that the reports are very conscientiously arrived at. Of forty pupils, hardly two or three have to have their categories reversed. There has been much controversy about the advantages and inconveniences of this division of classes into A and B, and it is difficult to pronounce a final judgement upon it. The good side of this institution is that it gives consideration to each child's rhythm of work, and that its intention is to create a more favourable atmosphere for study. The advanced pupil finds himself among his peers, and the weaker does not feel too much isolated since he is in the midst of comrades whose mental level is much the same as his own. Theoretically, then, it has the advantage of neither retarding the 'well-endowed' nor discouraging the hindmost. Cases have occurred in which a child who was among the lowest of Class A and was therefore demoted to Class B, has regained so much self-confidence that it has immediately risen to the head of its new class.

But this division does not present advantages only, and we wonder whether the objections are not more considerable. Is it not premature to decide so much of the future of a child of, at most, ten years? It is a decision pregnant with consequences, for by putting it into category B one debars it, almost certainly, from access to any liberal career. There are always some children who do not develop till the age of puberty. That will be too late and they will almost inevitably have to renounce the highest subjects of study. There is a no less evident injustice done to those whose assimilation of knowledge is slower, but who may be just as intelligent as their quicker schoolfellows. As an adaptation to the needs of the child, the merits of the arrangement are very relative, for it recognizes the individual's manner of working only by depriving him of future opportunities. Moreover, we have observed among many children of Class B an evident feeling of inferiority. Without knowing precisely upon what principle they have been classified, they frequently have a feeling that they have been numbered among those 'of whom not much is expected', and that all the brighter pupils are in the A classes. Such a feeling can in certain cases have objectionable consequences, for it is as dangerous continually to under-estimate as to over-esteem oneself.

Furthermore, we have often noticed a profound aversion between classes A and B, the children of the latter having a vague impression that something is being withheld from them and that those of the A classes enjoy better conditions. As for the A class pupils, they sometimes happen to preen themselves in the presence of their comrades of the other category, and between the two an unpleasant rivalry arises, exerting a pernicious influence upon the progress of both. It is true that the master counts for much in the opinions that the two groups entertain of one another, and this gave us a further opportunity to judge of the value of Adlerian psychology in practical education. This is, at bottom, against any principle of division, and would prefer a selective method which took no future possibility away from any child. Since however the school is obliged to conform to the general usage, it can only contrive arrangements that may make the best of it, seeking, e.g., for means of compensating any inferiority feelings engendered in Class B, and trying to transmute the latent rivalries into friendly emulation.

In support of what has just been said, we will cite one example among many that we recorded.

The children of the A classes were rehearsing a play of their own composition which was to be performed before the parents as a feature of a school festival. We happened by chance to come across some members of the B classes, all of whom appeared to be over-excited. The teacher of German, who worked in both divisions (the same subject is taught by the same master to all the classes, in accordance with the system of specialized instructors—the 'Fachlehrersystem'), did not show any surprise at this. The children then told him that they knew their more privileged schoolfellows were trying to write a play, and that they wanted to do as much themselves. Far from wishing to dissuade them, he adroitly directed them towards a subject that might well lend itself to their fantasy, while leaving it to them to choose an appropriate title. Their choice was finally fixed unanimously upon a mythological theme (Hercules at the crossroads), known to them all, which they intended to render in topical form by embodying their own experiences in it. For hours and hours, and with incredible enthusiasm, they worked on without relaxation, delighted to be engaged in the same work as the others whom they believed to be usually esteemed above them. Not one of them questioned for a moment the much greater difficulty of the A classes' undertaking. For the latter it was a case of completing their history course, according to their own expressed desire, by the writing of a drama upon the slave trade in ancient Greece.

The presentation that followed was equally enjoyable and successful on both sides. All had contributed to it in their various ways, either as authors, actors, decorators or stage hands. Thanks to this very simple and acceptable solution, one that followed the bent of the children's own interests, tension was thus transformed into happy emulation. All had been encouraged by experiencing the joy and expansion of success; and co-operation in a common purpose had been a strengthening exercise in interior discipline.

Adlerian method thus makes it possible to diminish the drawbacks of this separation of classes into disparate halves, which bears less hardly on the B pupils in the experimental school than in most of the other schools. This is made possible chiefly by the close collaboration of the masters. Each has formed the excellent habit of discussing, during the recreation period, what has been happening in the class he is about to teach. He is thus informed about the work the class has in hand, any unusual conduct on the part of one pupil or another; in short about the general mood of the class at that time. This very simple custom enables each master to get the best results with the least trouble and makes the work more enjoyable for everyone concerned.

It may not be without interest to mention an opinion that is held by the masters of the experimental school concerning the A and B classification, observing, however, that this opinion is only hypothetical and still wants confirmation. Dr. Spiel, for example, has the impression that the B classes are the better, both in class discipline and in their sense of community. For this rather surprising judgement he offers the following reasons: in the A divisions there is a certain rivalry, especially between the older pupils, who know that only the best of them will be admitted to college. They are animated by a personal interest, which is vital rather than egoistic, but from time to time it makes them forget their duties to their group. This would mean that they sometimes lose sight of the new, co-operative aim, forgetting to notice how they themselves are behaving; and the signs of a struggle for prestige at once emerge. The cleverer a child is the more duty it owes to the community: but it may take time—years, or even a whole life-time—to realize the fact. Not without justice, humanity expects more from one who is more favoured. To realize the truth of communal living, these children will have a harder task than their less brilliant comrades, who will serve that truth with fewer interior conflicts once they have recognized its grandeur. Must one infer, then, as Dr. Birnbaum does, that the behaviour varies inversely with the intelligence? Perhaps it does so in extreme cases, but not with the great majority. Without denying that a close relation exists between intelligence and character, one must beware of attempting any general definition. It is for the school to discern, in each case, how much help a pupil needs in order to attain his own equilibrium, and to occupy to the best possible advantage the position that falls to his lot.

The division into A and B is not, after all, of much danger to Adlerian classes, who may even use it to furnish additional evidence in favour of the ideas that inspire their work.

5. *Community of life and experience* (Erlebnisgemeinschaft)

By this we mean whatever draws the children together in a bond of feeling, whether it be a spectacle they all admire, a new invention they have just seen at an exhibition, and so forth. Do they not from time to time enjoy the incomparable pleasure of a journey together, of acquiring unforgettable memories in common? Does not the cinema screen often show them unknown countries in which they travel as though they were themselves the discoverers, triumphing over great obstacles? A sufficiency of such shared experience constitutes an essential factor in social education. In experiencing the same feelings as their comrades all become aware of a real community of life.

Let us briefly recapitulate this educational programme. Its object is, first, to form independent personalities, apt for co-operation and able to fulfil their duties towards humanity. The means adopted are limited communities, which together make up the great community of life of which all are members, children, parents and teachers.

In the *working community* the children learn together how to surmount the difficulties they will all have to encounter, to put forth the necessary efforts that duty may require of them. It is this that enables a child to develop all its faculties for its optimum performance.

Thanks to the *administrative community* they learn how to observe and to criticize with as much objectivity as possible.

By the *community of conversation* they learn how to listen to their neighbour, to judge of his argument while considering all the circumstances which have conditioned his behaviour. For it is difficult not to begin by unloading all one has on one's own heart, instead of first helping one's comrade by trying to understand *him*. It is perhaps in the course of these collective conversations that we could most readily recognize the educators of to-morrow. They furnish indications, at least, of fitness for the needs of the teaching vocation better than any arbitrary choice. The child who has learned to discern the motives and the consequences of its actions will be the most likely also to help its comrade to do the same. Every child needs thus to find the just measure between the feelings of relief it experiences in these conversations and the feelings of responsibility that they also induce.

The *community of mutual help* is that which prompts the child to be always ready to help its neighbour, as the most natural thing in the world.

Lastly, the *community of experience* is, as it were, the reward of the life lived in common. Everything here belongs to everyone, all pains are shared. But so are all the joys; as when the lights of the school festival seem to illuminate the very skies above these Viennese children, dispelling the gloom that too often darkens their little lives.

If, from this communal standpoint, we compare the ordinary State schools with the Adlerian experimental one, the conclusion is that the former try to make their working communities efficient means to instruction. On the other hand their communal administration is lax, incomplete or frankly non-existent. Communities of conversation and mutual help are unknown among them, save for rare exceptions, notably that of Fräulein Régine Seidler; some community of experience is however encouraged in all of them partly to supplement the teaching, and partly in order to give some recognition, after all, to a means of education otherwise neglected.

The experimental school, on the contrary, devotes every effort to its educational aim. Here the masters are always great friends with their boys. In all specially difficult or refractory cases they have recourse to the medico-pedagogic councils to which we shall refer later. This procedure almost always proves highly efficacious; leading to a change of atmosphere that is often in itself sufficient to dispel difficulties which shortly before had seemed insurmountable. Admittedly, this work of intimate collaboration, this common contribution of all towards the advent of a better world than this, is far from being perfectly achieved. It is the ideal, however, that they hold in mind, and strive with all their powers to realize as nearly as they can.

C. SYNTHESIS

We come now to the essential point of the Adlerian school. Most of the public schools we visited are committed to the reformed method of instruction; they attribute the greatest importance to this and their interest in educational problems is but slight. At the beginning of the reform there were indeed teachers who did not neglect the latter aspect of their work. But since both successes and failures of instruction were of so much official importance, and the masters usually so dependent upon them, it is not surprising that the majority of these educators have yielded pride of place to the aim of instruction. They are therefore led to pay only so much attention to the educational ideal as may be useful to instruction. Moreover, they may be somewhat discouraged. Feeling isolated in their concern for essential education and afraid of risking their position if they wander from the beaten track, they have to renounce their aspirations and submit to the official requirements. Collaboration alone can ensure the victory of an idea; the isolated advocate is courting certain defeat.

Faithful to Dr. Adler's principles, the experimental

school has drawn from them a power to survive successive periods of crisis. Its constant preoccupation has been to achieve a living synthesis of teaching with education. It would be no more satisfied with the most perfect education pursued apart from teaching, than it is with instruction given regardless of the character of the child.

No hard and fast line can be drawn between the requirements of teaching and of education, two aspects of the problem which should never be separated in practice; the Adlerian teacher in fact does all he can to fill the gap between them. The experimental school method tends therefore to look something like a synthesis of the methods of Dr. Decroly, de Ferrière and of Dr. Montessori. Its insistence upon collective activity recalls the activism of the great Belgian educationist, who so well understood its efficacy in stimulating the child's will to acquire knowledge. In availing itself to the utmost of the principles of the active school, the experimental school reminds one of de Ferrière; and finally, following the example of the great Italian teacher, it seeks to develop the senses of the child by individual activity. Now, the 'active school', instead of trying, as in times past, to inculcate the maximum amount of knowledge (Lernschule) preoccupies itself with the pupil's productivity and initiative. What it wants is to see the child learning to set problems to itself. The experimental school tries to go a step beyond this; its aim is to become 'a school of rôles' (Birnbaum's 'Rollenschule') which means that the child actually 'plays a part' varying with the subject in hand: it sets itself, for instance, actually to be a physicist when it is studying physics; a traveller or an explorer when it is learning geography. To enable children to play these rôles, proper equipment is of course necessary—for the sciences, a physical laboratory; for geography, a room with pictures and photographs of various countries, and above all a large sand relief (Birnbaum speaks of the 'Reizwelt'). The laboratories made us think of the Dalton Laboratory Plan, but that would not really suffice, for it pays too little attention to collective activity. According to Adler himself, the system of Winnetka comes nearest to his idea, because it takes into consideration both the child's individual performance—postulating a minimum schedule of information each child has to acquire—and the collective performance, to which half the time is devoted. However, without recourse to Winnetka's ingenious system, one can apply the Adlerian principles from day to day, without any change of equipment or any expense. It is enough if the masters have the root of the matter in them. Their successes will not then be long delayed.

Autodidacticism[1] and *co-operation* are the two complementary ideals that the experimental school has set itself, and the nearer it attains to them, the worthier will be the citizens that it produces.

By co-operation the child develops its feeling of solidarity with others whilst by autodidactic action it strengthens its individuality. Step by step as it improves in both respects, it overcomes its errors and becomes more clearly a personality accountable for its own past, present and future, with a wholeness that enables it to avail itself of all its powers. For a past of which one does not feel acquitted always operates as an inhibition in the present. The child needs to utter the courageous 'yes' that is an affirmation equally of what is good in it and what is bad, before it says the 'and yet' which is an impulse to persevere, unfavourable though the immediate conditions may appear. The first stage is that of recognizing and understanding one's mistakes; the second, that of confessing them; then and not before, a fresh

---

[1] We apologise for reproducing this term for which we can find no satisfactory equivalent; including as it does the ideas of self-criticism and self-training—Trans.

affirmation becomes possible, one that may lay the foundation of a new life, lived in view of the community.[1] It is the putting into practice of the Socratic 'know thyself'.

We have already touched upon the question of *talents* or gifts (Begabungen). Many teachers and parents are quick to ascribe any striking success in whatever kind of work to an exceptional talent, and are equally prone to explain set-backs as due to lack of talent. In support of this view they cite all the child's forebears, gifted or otherwise in the same direction. In mathematics especially, they presume quite hastily to judge of a child's talent; and even while they allow that the master and the method may have contributed much to a given result, they never fail to find the final explanation in the presence or absence of talent. But is any question more delicate than this of *talent*? How is it that a child that was a dunce at a particular subject suddenly displays talent in it; or, on the other hand, that a child which has shown a marked facility loses it, after changing over to a new teacher, for instance? The mysterious thing that we call 'talent', 'gift' or 'aptitude' but never manage to define satisfactorily—does it not amount, after all, to a kind of courage, of perseverance in training, as Adlerian psychology considers it? True, an Adlerian teacher, though he puts no faith in talent, does not categorically deny its existence. He prefers to admit our theoretical ignorance upon this point, and in practice to act on the principles he has espoused. His reduction of 'talent' to a development in the earliest years, under certain conditions of encouragement and training, serves him as a working hypothesis, of proven fruitfulness in many cases. Moreover, it much enlarges the field of action for the teacher who adopts it.

As we have seen, Adlerian psychology envisages all psychic manifestations from a finalist standpoint. Thus, in

[1] Cf. Kunkel's concepts: Einsicht, Eingeständnis, Bejahung.

the presence of a lazy or backward pupil (setting aside cases of idiocy or feeble-mindedness) it looks first of all to see what the child effects by laziness, feigned stupidity or lack of aptitude. For it considers that such attitudes may be *measures of security* (Sicherungen) unconsciously adopted by the child. These subterfuges excuse it from effectual effort by enabling it to escape from any sense of responsibility. In every idler the Adlerian sees a discouraged individual—unless, of course, he is suffering from an organic illness.

Many people, when they look for the causes of laziness in a child, try to trace them back to hereditary factors. Unfortunately, a child who sees that its elders have discovered a reason for it to be idle will feel reinforced in its behaviour and make no further effort to change. Is it not much simpler to fall back upon this fictitious excuse than to go forward and risk a set-back amongst its comrades? Nor is it otherwise with the children supposed to be stupid or incapable. They are constantly preoccupied with measures of insurance against having to enter the arena of life, always seeking a dispensation from responsibility. But children that have neither successes nor defeats to their name can come to no good. Nor is it at all surprising when we see them trying, by delinquent behaviour, to give themselves a false importance.

We have already observed that the teacher has to gain the child's confidence, in order to discover its plan of life and enable it to understand, in appropriate terms, the error of its ways. Then only can he undertake the re-education of one who has been expending his energies to no purpose. Since this is done simply with a view to eliminating future mistakes, the prognosis must naturally be optimistic. The child will then feel that the teacher has no desire whatever to condemn his behaviour, but only to make him able to improve it. Knowing that the first step is always the most costly to take, the educator will offer the little one a helping hand, and try to put it in the way of gaining some initial success. For this he will have recourse to the intimate collaboration of the parents and his colleagues, which alone makes such re-educative care possible.

D. EXAMPLES OF COLLECTIVE CONVERSATION
(Klassenbesprechungen)

To demonstrate the application of this synthesis of instruction and education, let us now give a few examples. All the pupils are assembled before the master and one of his colleagues: the head boy reads the agenda for the day drawn up in collaboration with all the others. Whoever has a desire to say something makes it known to the head of the class, so that it may be entered in the agenda. The session is thus opened, and the head boy asks the leader of each group in turn what he thinks about its members. Some leaders declare themselves satisfied, others consider that the performance of their group might have been better. In the latter case, the group-members themselves may perhaps protest that their leader is too severe, and try to persuade him that they would obey him better if he led them in a friendlier manner. Here are some of the points raised in the course of collective discussion. (1) The head boy (2) the savings-box for an excursion (3) the bad behaviour of certain pupils during the gymnastics period. It rather frequently happens that the discussion of the first question raised is so prolonged that no time remains for the others.

Here is a collective conversation that took place between the youngest pupils (ten years of age) on the subject of *discipline*. Knowing as they do so little about it, it is not surprising that they very often return to this question. The class is upon the point of electing its head boy.

(*M.* = master, *P.* = one or other of the pupils.)

M. How shall we do this?

P. By having an election.

M. Of course, but we haven't got to that yet. What kind of boy is wanted for a head boy?

P. He should have a good character.

M. Why?

P. So that he can always set us a good example. And he ought to be strong; we want to be able to cheek him if we like and he won't lose his temper.

P. He should be like a master because he takes the master's place.

M. And what else ought he to be?

P. He needs to speak well so that he can always speak up for our class.

P. He needs to be just.

The pupils propose a head boy, but one of them objects that the candidate is not sufficiently robust.

P. But why does our leader have to be strong? The general of an army needn't be the strongest man in it. What is important is that he should have brains in his head.

P. I agree with what has just been said, but I don't agree about the boy they propose. He's too calm, too quiet.

P. That's not fair. When you first came you had still less to say for yourself than X. He hasn't been with us long. He has first to get used to all the boys. No more does a machine work its best from the very beginning. You have to get to know all about it first.

During the election the boy proposed is sent out of the room, so that he may not know which of his companions have voted for or against him. He is chosen by a large majority of the class. The master then explains in a few words what are the difficulties of being head boy and the responsibilities of that position, and asks everyone to co-operate peaceably in the communal life that they are about to make for themselves. Later, he takes the new head boy aside to explain more of the nature of his function and authorizes him to visit another class, where a head boy has been elected some time ago, and to join it in a collective conversation.

At another session, the class spent its time in working out for itself the rules it was to observe in the course of collective conversation. This class had indeed suffered enough from disorder to feel the need for rules that everyone would respect. The children finally came to agreement upon the following:

(1) Whoever is speaking must be allowed to finish what he is saying.

(2) There must be no shouting, for no one will be listened to any the better for it.

(3) Whoever is speaking must be listened to by everyone.

(4) Only the speaker must stand, the rest must stay in their seats.

(5) The speaker who speaks next must go on from what the last speaker has just said.

(6) If anyone holds up his hand he is to be allowed to speak at once.

The last rule is really made for the timid pupils, who lack the courage simply to get up and speak when they have something to say. It is a device that may draw them into discussion. Among the timid there are, of course, some who are very content to say nothing from lack of interest. But they will soon be found out, and for their special benefit this last rule was established:

(7) Everyone must say something at least once in the hour.

These disciplinary rules are respected with a rigour and conscientiousness that could not possibly be obtained for regulations arbitrarily imposed by the master. Autonomy is undoubtedly the best instrument of education, and it belongs to the art of the educator to lead the child to do its duties of its own free will.

A point of importance in this connexion is that the same master is in charge of the same pupils throughout the whole of the school period of four years. He therefore gets to know each one very well, and the influence he has upon them is the more efficacious for being of adequate duration.

Here, now, is a collective conversation which is concerned above all with the *combative instinct*.

To understand what a critical question this may become in the experimental school, one must remember that the children have nowhere to disport themselves during their periods of recreation. They are obliged to spend them in class, where they cannot run and gambol around as children need to do: since the school is without means to relieve this privation, the pupils have to accommodate themselves to a condition which the masters accept only under protest.

The first point on the agenda for this day is as follows:

Why one often wants to fight
(*von der wiederaufsteigenden Rauflust*)

P. I think there is a likeness between enjoying a fight and the pleasure of having an argument. And because the strong are always being teased by the weak they quite naturally want to fight.

M. Do you think that only the strong have the right to fight—or what do you think about it?

Several pupils at once. No. That wouldn't be fair!

P. Anyway, it's the strongest who have been using that right for some time here.

84

P. Perhaps that's only a passing thing, and the combative instinct will calm down in time.

M. Well, then, shall we just fold our arms and wait till that time comes? That would be convenient and effective.

What do you think? Some of you may perhaps convince me that children should be allowed to fight when they want to. After all I have nothing against a little battle between friends. It is rather pleasant to exercise one's strength. There are reasons, however, why we can't have you fighting one another in class.

P. I've noticed that it's always the same ones who begin it . . .

It is noteworthy that no names are mentioned. This anonymity is meant primarily to exclude from these discussions any thought of being 'reported'. Those whose conduct is mentioned know very well who is being referred to.

P. Whoever wants a fight will only go for another fighter. A comrade who wouldn't hit him back doesn't interest him at all. What matters to him is not so much to hurt anyone as to find an enemy. To be able to fight there must be two.

As soon as the boy has said those words the master writes them on the blackboard—'To be able to fight there must be two'. This is a method often used by the teachers at the experimental school in the course of collective conversations. Every point arrived at in common is noted on the blackboard, so that everyone can see where the discussion has got to. It helps in keeping the argument consecutive and the pupils learn to think more correctly.

P. There is one among us who never wants to fight. We all know that he never hits back, and we hardly ever cheek him.

This refers to John, a good pupil of average ability. He is a serious child, of very frank character, much respected by all the class. After a few moments' silence, a pupil puts this question:

P. Why does nobody want to fight John? I may as well give his name as we all know he is the one, besides, we're not blaming him . . .

P. We all know he won't fight, so it isn't worth while.

P. I believe John never did want to fight. He's not aggressive and gets no pleasure out of it.

M. But there's more to say about John. You have not yet got to the bottom of this question. I rather feel that you hesitate to go on with it for fear that you might have to draw conclusions disagreeable or painful to some of you.

P. I believe John doesn't fight because he's clever.

M. Indeed he is an intelligent pupil, I wouldn't say more than that. But let each one draw the consequences on his own account. I fancy that if you think of John next time you are starting a fight you will perhaps have quite a new feeling about it.

P. This makes me think of our history lesson. Caesar was the best for having ideas, Crassus for carrying them out.

M. It seems to me that it is present circumstances that remind you of those things of 2,000 years ago. When anyone feels uncomfortable in the present, he gladly escapes into the past.

At this the children perceive that they are trying to evade something. It is therefore a propitious moment for them to go forward and learn something more.

M. Let everyone now look into himself.

P. I think John is good, and that is why he feels no need to fight better than the others.

P. We don't separate boys into good and bad here. We think children are just intelligent or stupid.

M. What kind of feelings do you have for a child like John, who never gets into a temper when he is teased?

The first answer takes a little while to come.

P. I believe I know why so many boys are always wanting to fight. They think they will never be 'top dog' at anything else, so they want at least to be the best fighters. It's as though they chose an easier way.

Note the perspicacity with which these children judge one another!

P. There can be two kinds of victory: one in fighting with your fists and the other in struggling with your mind.

M. Think of Gandhi who never gives in, who never rebels and who refuses to fight the English. How, for all that, can he be known and esteemed all over the world?

P. It's his mind that makes us respect him.

P. We all feel admiration for Gandhi. So do I for John, too.

The teacher writes on the board the word *admiration*. He is about to turn the conversation in such a way as to relieve the situation for little John who has for some time been feeling ill at ease. It is risky to heap praises upon a child because it is always difficult to make him accept them in the right way, and the master does not want the conversation to end upon this note.

M. Since John is an intelligent boy, he cares little about being admired. He would do no more and no less to get the admiration of anyone. But what he does like is to be respected. That is why I believe he will go on doing his duty as he has done up to the present, and that you will continue to respect him, and draw from this conversation conclusions that apply to yourselves.

P. (in a loud voice). We ought to do like him.

The conversation being over, several children set upon John to tease him, half in friendly fun, but partly by pretending to be really hostile. They want to test this goodness of his, but they feel more like hugging him than hurting him. Thus the master has succeeded in calming their minds and at the same time has put John down from a rather dangerous prominence to the place where he belongs. No harm will have been done to him by this discussion, and the majority of his school-mates will have learnt an unforgettable lesson from it.

We now turn to the *sexual problem*, which occupies quite a special place in the Viennese schools, and in the experimental school which, in this respect, has to conform to the rest. In theory, there is no such problem, since the teachers are strictly forbidden to mention it. Neither in the course of the natural science lessons nor in collective or mutual conversations have the teachers a right to explain anything at all in this domain of sex, which is reserved for the parents. The prohibition is a serious obstacle to education, for sexual training is an integral part of it. Indeed, it seems rather paradoxical that the Viennese schools, in general so advanced, should have entirely banned sexual education from their syllabus. However that may be, this regulation is rigorously maintained and anyone transgressing it risks his situation. The masters in the experimental school are the worst sufferers since their ideal is to give the children as complete an education as possible, and at the present time parents are nearly all incapable of giving a child the sexual education which is their exclusive prerogative. If they are informed neither at school nor at home, the children very naturally have recourse to those older companions who 'know something' already. That this is not the best kind of initiation into the facts of life has to be admitted. Others prefer to seek the satisfaction of their curiosity in a special kind of literature, a procedure which is hardly better than the former but rather worse. All that the teachers can do, when they see that a child is continually pre-occupied with questions of this nature, is to call in the mother and advise her to speak to her child. As this is generally ineffectual they but rarely resort to it. To the teachers in the Adlerian school, indeed, there is one way only to remedy this important defect—that is, to work for such a well-balanced development of the child that it will be able to look after itself in the sexual sphere, without prejudice to what the school strives constantly to teach him; the respect due to others and to himself.

This deficiency in the reform of the Viennese schools is all the more regrettable because no one would be better qualified than the Adlerian psychologists for initiating children into the sexual problem. Moreover, the children perceive very well that there are certain subjects which, even in this school, are not to be entered upon. Conse-quently these things inevitably acquire the attraction of forbidden fruit and tend to capture the child's special atten-tion, unless it strives scrupulously to repress all spontaneity about them. Never quite managing thus to free its mind from what is bound to appear so 'vile' that it must not be even mentioned, a child sometimes suffers from a feeling of guilt that hinders its normal development. Such an arrange-ment takes no account of the natural interest of the young in the sexual question. There is no need for astonishment if children betray their desire to acquire some information upon this subject, even if they do so in ways not very wel-come to their teachers. At the experimental school there are still, unavoidably, some masters who have but imperfectly assimilated the ideas of Dr. Adler, and it is from them that the boys instinctively try to get information. They know very well that it annoys these masters, which makes the subject all the more intriguing. A class has been known to arrange, just before the lesson in religious knowledge, to ask several 'posers' one after another, all touching upon sexuality. In this way they could turn the religious lesson into an entertainment, and torment the teacher by their attempts to penetrate a little into this domain of adult secrets. Their questions were, indeed, very innocent and infantile. They asked, for instance, whether it was possible, as they had read in a book, for children living on an island to have babies.

One day, the children carried things to such a point that the lesson became impossible, but one of them rebelled and spoke to the master of the class about it. It was in the month of February when the certificates had just been distributed, and to their surprise most of the children had done badly in religion. To this many of them attached little importance because they thought, as their parents did, that religious knowledge was no longer essential in the modern world. But the master, who knew better, pointed out their mistake. He called their attention to a growing tendency amongst employers, when choosing apprentices, to inquire not only how many marks they had for conduct but also for religion, which they now looked upon as complementary and necessary. Then he tried to make them understand that their attitude was wanting in refinement and unworthy of big boys for whom the experimental school was taking so much trouble. Were they really unable to adapt themselves, even for one subject, to a thing they disliked?

Hitherto, during the religious lessons, one pupil had been appointed as a supervisor, and he had to report those who behaved badly, so that they could be spoken to in the course of the collective discussions. After this exhortation from the teacher, however, the pupils suddenly found this procedure disagreeable and unsatisfactory. Something had changed in them, and they wanted the police measure abolished. They even went so far as vehemently to criticize the conduct of the boy who had warned the master of the class, denouncing him as a spy and an informer. But the master then asked them:

'On the other hand, did it not take some courage for him to be the first to pull himself up on the bad road taken by the whole class?' Rather than treat him as an informer, ought they not to thank him, for having brought the class back to ways more worthy of it? One of the pupils then declared that he, too, was sure that the boy in question was not an informer: for a spy, he said, is one who goes secretly to work exploring something for the benefit of someone else. Since their schoolfellow had acted on his own initiative and only to be of use to those he 'reported', he had really behaved with intelligence and bravery.

To end this discussion, the master told the story of a mayor who had been disliked by the government because he brought many scandals to light.

'. . . Nothing escaped him. He feared nothing when the need was to speak the truth. No sumptuous monument has been erected to him, but he knew how to win over the hearts of men. For his uprightness he was loved and respected by the people, and although this admirable man was never awarded decorations, he will always live in the mind of the masses. You see, then, how unpleasant it may be to put things in their true light and how much courage it needs to do so, for one who unmasks abuses is seldom liked. But as you have just seen, such a man is not to be compared with a spy, on the contrary he is the true servant of the common good. Think about that. I can see we are already beginning to understand one another better . . .'

On another occasion, when we were present, the conversation in common was about starting a *savings-bank* to finance a school excursion. This was a most animated discussion, for everyone had to be enabled to join in this outing, else it could not take place. How were they to get the necessary money?

Some proposed a box hung upon the wall, in which each one was to put as many halfpennies as he could. They wanted, very democratically, to see the same amount of pleasure for everyone arranged by mutual aid, so that no one should feel inferior. But there was quite a party against this point of view. These were afraid that some well-to-do pupil might, in an evil hour, make the poorer ones feel that they could only join in the school journey thanks to his pennies. Finally the children came to agreement upon the creation of two boxes; a regular box into which everyone would put what he could each week, and have it entered by the responsible cashier in the savings-book; and another box for voluntary 'gifts'. In this way each pupil would know what he had deposited, and the contents of the two boxes were to be combined at the last moment to make up the common purse. It is a point of some interest that hardly any child brought more than a halfpenny a week. Many of them indeed brought nothing for months, either because their parents could not spare them a single halfpenny or— as we learnt later was not uncommon—because they spent their halfpennies on a more immediate pleasure, such as a visit to the cinema. It is not surprising to find such an attitude widespread among the young, especially among these children who had seen their parents losing from day to day all that they had saved for years past. In their impoverished existence, such children do not know how to resist the desire to give themselves a pleasure as soon as ever they have the means. Their excursion money-box filled up very slowly: but what could one expect of little people whose lives were passed in such penury?

We shall see in due course what happened about this savings-bank question some weeks later.

One day the children learnt that a *secret society* had been formed in the very bosom of the class. This discovery aroused a regular revolution. Everyone was speaking at once, hot tempers were rising and the six members of the secret society were indignantly denounced as traitors to the community of the class. We found that these six were among the most intelligent boys in the class, who were banded together to make some additional savings in order to help a comrade who was especially hard up. The whole affair had remained secret until the moment when they thought fit to expel one of their members, whom they no longer thought worthy of their confidence. It was he who had 'split' upon the others.

W. (a member of the society). When we formed our association we promised each other to keep it secret. But now that the whole class knows about it we must tell them what has happened. We joined together to save money, so that our schoolmate D. could afford to be one of us. When we started our society he hadn't yet put in a single halfpenny and we decided to club together to help him. So you see we've done nothing wrong and you've nothing to get excited about.

P. To form societies like that doesn't seem to me a good thing, because it's going behind the backs of other boys who might have wanted to join in. That's not to the good of the community. It ought to be forbidden . . . but that's not right either, because they would be able to go on meeting outside the school and our community would suffer just as much.

W. Why, of course, if you won't allow it in class, we are still free to do it outside.

B. Do you think that's the way to make a proper community of the class? You've even got a secret writing, and you're always being seen whispering together about something. You're beginning to form a separate group which won't be about the savings-box alone, but against the good feeling of the class. It's a danger to all of us.

I. (a member of the society shouting passionately). Look here, what harm have we done to anybody? You are now turning things round as though we had some evil purpose!

—Not so loud! cry several at once.

I. You're making this very simple thing into some shocking story, a mystery!

While the children are getting heated again the master, who has not stirred a finger till now, writes the following words on the blackboard:

Community = an association for all
Secret Society; for mutual
aid = an association for some
What is there for it, and what against it?

M. We have at last happily arrived at the real point. You may now calm yourselves. I ought to confess to you that I have myself been a member of a secret society. But then the circumstances were different because we had no such thing as a class community; and I would have you know that if such societies have their good side they may also be a great danger. This must be reckoned with. Those who have been only listeners up to the present will now give us their opinions, for we want everyone's views, on this subject.

I. I do think, boys, you ought to make us understand, what is wrong about our society. If we can see that your arguments are right, we shall be ready to give in.

It is really extraordinary to see boys of ten and eleven showing so much mutual respect.

P. The first thing wrong that we have to blame you for is that the society is secret. If it is really good for everyone there's no need to hide it up as if it were the biggest mystery in the world.

C. If the chief aim is really to save up money, I can't see why you don't want everyone in it. If all thirty-six of us take part in it, that will bring in more than you who are only six.

The master, without a word, writes on the board:

36 is more than 6

An unquestionable mathematical fact!

F. (a member). Before Christmas, we all decided to save up together, so that everyone could go on the excursion. Well now, I ask you; what have you done since? What have you given up for it? Have you made, every now and then, the very little sacrifice that our community asked for, for the good of us all in the end? You haven't done anything at all and the box is still nearly empty now in March! If we had preferred to trust to you, we should never go on an excursion all our lives. That is why we clubbed together in secret to get some money saved.

M. It is the turn of the others to speak. The members' opinions are now known.

G. I think they are acting against the community.

While the children very eagerly carry on the discussion, the master writes on the blackboard:

THE ADLERIAN EXPERIMENTAL SCHOOL

Personal interest	General interest
Secret Society	*Community of the Class*

H. If you want an aim to succeed, everyone has to help in it. The scientific men have to work openly together; if not, they would never invent anything more.

L. But there's all the difference between a friend one can work with and a secret group.

Only at this point did the children notice what was written on the blackboard. There was a sudden silence. No one ventured to break it, since each of them guessed that his arguments might be only personal.

M. The debate has stopped all at once, because you all see how hard it is to argue without using the personal pronoun 'I'. But it is only objective arguments that count.

I. Does the society hurt the class? Are we taking anything away from you?

B. The purpose of your society is less to collect money than to look like heroes. You want the glory of having made it possible for D. to have the outing.

W. What an idea! If we'd wanted to swank we would have talked about the society. You're not saving anything. It seems unfair to us when one brings only a few halfpennies and another several shillings.

G. That's going back to personal things instead of telling us facts.

The way some of these children bring a schoolfellow back to the point at issue is remarkable. They show a sense of debating procedure that not a few parliaments might envy them!

Z. We're saving for D. and not for ourselves. If one day we have too much money we will all six go to the cinema. We don't need to save up for three jackets if D. needs only

96

one. I tell you that so that you may see that we're more like a party of good friends than a secret society, the thing you hate so much.

While the boys are discussing whether 'society' or 'party of friends' is the appropriate name for the secret arrangement that troubles them so much the master calls their ironical attention to the following circumstance:

There is a danger. There might be too much money.

N. I see quite another danger. If these boys begin going to the cinema together, they'll perhaps soon be asking their parents for money for the savings-bank but spending it for their own amusement. Or, if they really do want to beat us all by the amount they save, they'll perhaps have to do I don't know what to get hold of all the money they will need.

W. That's enough now. We've told you everything. Tell us if you please, yes or no, shall we six go on saving together in class. If you don't agree, I warn you in advance that we shall do it outside the school.

Several pupils. We want to work all together; we want all to save up for what we need.

F. (a member). What we do outside the school is no one's business. There we needn't pay attention to any community.

M. (turning to his colleague). Here is the first civil war. We are witnessing the first 'class struggle', in both senses of the word.

It is a fact of some interest that children in their third year of High School (their seventh year of schooling) nearly always rebel, at some point, against the community of the class. This community appears too narrow to some of them, and they begin suddenly to resent it as a restriction upon their personal liberty. These communities constitute, indeed, real, living organisms, passing through all the phases of evolution and abrupt change—that is, of revolution. It is almost always the most intelligent members of the class who suddenly begin a struggle for prestige against their comrades of yesterday. A fresh adaptation then becomes necessary; a new, internal transformation is needed if those who are trying to escape from the community are to become re-adapted to it. For the child of greater intelligence ought not to be privileged above its less advanced comrades; it has no less duty to live in harmony with all of them. The formation of minor groups within the community represents a danger to the community feeling which it is so important for the children to cultivate, if they are to grow up to be men capable of sacrifice for their neighbours.

Z. Why don't you want us to put all our savings together?

M. The society claims that it wants to come to the aid of D.

The Class. Yes, and that's right.

M. If I rightly understand what you have just said, I think you will have to draw the consequences. According to everyone of you, what you have at heart is to collect as much money as possible for D.

X. But all the boys must give to it. Only if they do, shall we manage to save all we can. If we ever saved more money than was needed, we would be able to go somewhere further away or to stay there longer.

W. (a member). This isn't fair at all, for you've been trying to save ever since Christmas; and you've never economized as much as we have, though we're only six, in three weeks! Let's try the experiment again: you economize all you can for three weeks. We'll do the same on our side, and we'll soon see who will have saved the most.

M. We've already exceeded our time; nevertheless, before we separate for to-day we must come to some decision. Now, think about this (and the master writes on the board):

$$\left.\begin{array}{c} \textit{Money from the class} \\ + \\ \textit{Money from the society} \end{array}\right\} \text{for D.}$$

L. Perhaps the best would be to have both the community and the society. We should then get a bigger amount.

M. Yes, and on the morning of the excursion, you would call in your school-mate D. and say, 'Open your hands'. In the right, he would receive the money from the class; in the left, the money from the society. But would a gift like that really please you?

N. That's not a good way. He ought to receive in both hands at once both the sum collected by the class and what the society collects.

I. (a member). We don't agree to do it that way. We don't want the moneys mixed together.

M. What do you think is at the bottom of that? What really is the desire that pushes you to help your school-mate. Is it a purely unselfish regard for D.?

B. What is pushing them most of all is the wish to out-shine us, not to help him.

M. This question about money for D. has raised as it were a wall around you all. You are all thus far taking too narrow or too short a view. Try to make out, on the other side of this wall, the real motive for what this group is doing.

P. It's ambition.

B. I propose we set up several little groups and that each one saves separately.

C. I don't agree. That would be the end of all community in our class.

D. I believe the society is putting money on one side to be able to spend it later on their own pleasure. That's a bad thing.

Members. Tell us, then: do you want our society dissolved?

X. We want all to give to the savings fund together.

M. It seems to me useless for you, feeling as you do, to decide upon any plan whatever. You are too excited to arrive at anything that will satisfy you when you have recovered your calm; and you would be unlikely to carry out any decision you would be able to make.

H. I propose we vote.

Class. No, that's no good!

W. (a member). Well, then, let's forbid our society! It will never again set itself up against the interests of the class, and we will do nothing more of the kind in school.

M. I fancy that the proposal made by W. doesn't please everybody.

B. No, because it's unsociable.

O. They will go on in just the same way outside school, and the community of our class will not suffer any less for that.

M. If you wish to try . . .

Several boys. No, no!

B. There would be bickering without any end.

E. Let's hang up a box over there and all put several halfpennies into it regularly.

M. To me it seems that you are bringing the class-struggle into the school. (The allusion was to what the class had learnt from history about the fierce struggle between the plebeians and the patricians in ancient Rome. And indeed, the six members of this secret society belonged almost wholly to the bourgeoisie, whilst the majority of the others were working-class children. As we noted, too, the intelligence and development of the six defendants was above the average. It would of course be wrong to draw any conclusion from these circumstances, but it cannot be denied that an easy and cultivated home exerts a favourable influence upon a child's progress both physical and mental.)

P. Yes, like it was in Rome between the plebeians and the aristocrats.

Members. All right, if you don't want us any more, we'll simply go into another class.

E. Do as you like; you're absolutely free.

W. (a member: abruptly rising). I believe I've found out what is at the bottom of this question. This community in class, which we all want, does it have to be kept up just as much outside school? It seems to me everything depends on that.

E. We're not interested in what they do outside school. They can do what they want to.

M. My friends, I shall say no more about this for to-day. There is evidently something important you have not yet realized. Do you believe there is a limit to the sacrifices that one ought to make for the common good? After all, if someone asks you whether he ought not to practise the community of the class just as much outside the class, isn't it because he finds it more comfortable to do what he wants to first, before serving his neighbour? Think about that for next time.

In this way the moment has come for the master to pass his pupils on from the community of the class-room to the common life at large. This animated discussion shows us that they are capable of surmounting the barriers that appeared to exist between the one and the other. Perhaps their whole being will be changed by the new truth of which they have just become aware: There is no limit to one's duty towards the community, for that duty may widen out to infinity.

We have preserved this collective conversation because it enables us to illustrate two points of interest.

(1) The recognition by these children that the duty the individual owes to the community is without limits.

(2) Their complete inability to effect personal economies, after what their families have suffered in the recent social upheavals.

We saw more than one class, which had achieved good internal discipline and was living in excellent harmony with its teachers, show itself incapable of making the smallest efforts to save up for a school excursion. Unless the master himself took trouble about it, nothing was done to fill the savings-box, although everyone wanted very much to join in the proposed excursion. Even the efforts of the master himself were often fruitless, for the children would simply declare that they did not possess a penny, and one had to appeal to the parents' association.

In reality, nearly all Viennese children spend their pocket-money upon immediate pleasures. That incontinent habit is widespread among the mass of the people and the teachers do all that they can to counteract it. They try to cultivate in these children the strength to give up a cinema from time to time for a future advantage which, by an error of perspective, seems to them smaller.

This mentality prevails everywhere. By way of example, here is a collective conversation at which we were present in one of the ordinary schools, that of Fräulein Seidler, the disciple of Dr. Adler whom we have already had occasion to mention. Her position is extremely difficult, since she is the only one in her school to put Adlerian ideas into practice. She nevertheless obtains remarkable results in her class, which consists of between thirty and forty little girls. With a rare psychological insight, she conducts their education thinking of them all the time as the young mothers of to-morrow, the educators of the next generation.

One Monday morning Fräulein Seidler had the idea of asking her pupils how they had spent their Sunday, since the majority of them had professed themselves unable to find the small annual subscription (of 80 Groschen) that would admit them to the sessions for planning school outings which form a highly instructive adjunct to the lessons in geography. The parents' association comes to the aid of the children who cannot afford this, a support upon which they are all too willing to lean. Some twenty of these girls of thirteen or fourteen years of age had spent their afternoon at the cinema, at the theatre or at a children's dance. But here are their own reports:

D. I had been ill all the week. So I felt I had a good right to give myself a little treat and go to the cinema on Sunday.

R. I can't possibly stay in the house on Sunday: what do you expect me to do? Why, I go to the cinema; besides that's the best fun there is.

A. When I've worked all through the week, I must go to see and hear something else on Sunday.

And when the mistress suggests that they might at least go to see instructional films, they exclaim that these are too dull, and remind them too much of school. What they look for on Sundays is a diversion that will be a complete change from what they do in the week.

Poor children! It is their everyday unhappiness that makes them so avid for pleasure. Whatever can make them forget their life, presents an irresistible attraction. But though we understand, one must not yield to them on this point; to do so would not make for their future happiness, but the reverse.

Here is another example, this one relating to a *border-line case*.

Adlerian psychology makes no pretension that it is able to reconcile every difficult child to society. When a child's behaviour is symptomatic of a progressive mental disease, the Adlerian knows no more than any other psychotherapy how to prevent it. But even here it is distinguished among other psychologies by its readiness to try everything in a doubtful case, shrinking from no sacrifice so long as the doctors hesitate before an adverse diagnosis. Only in the gravest of cases, where the medical prognosis is entirely unfavourable, does the Adlerian consent to withdraw the child from its social and educational situation and have it interned in a sanatorium.

The example is of a boy of thirteen, E., who has just been entered in the third class of the experimental school, that which corresponds to his age. He has already passed through five schools and institutions, has even been for a time at Eggenburg (a great re-educational centre to which only the most difficult children are admitted). Nowhere have they been able to keep him, so aggressive is he towards both masters and school-mates. He cannot be left for an instant without supervision, lest he should break everything within his reach or attack another child and beat it up. Upon his entry into the experimental school he replies with blows when his class-mates ask him what school he came from (a favourite question when entering into contact with a new pupil) and he gives the same treatment to anyone who asks where he lives. We had never seen such a little volcano: another eruption was to be feared at any moment.

As one may imagine, it was no joke for a class to have to

put up with such a personality. His presence was a heavy burden, but everyone applied himself with unbelievable patience to conciliate the irascible E. However, there is always a limit, and a moment came when the entire class turned against him. This was a regular revolution, which of course changed nothing. In despair of the case, the masters tried out several stratagems. For instance, they told E. to supervise the corridors during recreation, for then the children have the class-rooms to themselves, and it is the masters themselves who walk about in the corridors. Or they entrusted him with a notebook in which he was to write down any good thing he saw in his schoolfellows. But from the first day of this he recorded nothing but faults and never ceased to disparage the others.

One pupil in the class wanted to try to become E.'s friend. He felt no liking for him, but wished to make the sacrifice because he felt it was the only way of gaining the little rebel's confidence. With admirable perseverance he kept constantly near him, and always took his part against the class. All went well for a few days, but it was only a treacherous calm before the next tempest which soon broke out.

The last method was then resorted to. The child was isolated in the master's office and kept at work there to accustom him to the master. Even with everyone's collaboration, this effort proved unavailing. In the end, E. began to bite his schoolfellows so savagely that their parents demanded his immediate expulsion.

E.'s parents had not the means to have him placed in a 'home' where Adlerian methods are applied to extremely a-social children. Nor had he the right to enter another school, having already attended six schools in vain.

Here, then, is the case of a child whose intellect appears to be sound (his school work was excellent) but whose malicious behaviour makes him socially intolerable. He will remain upon his parents' hands, until one day he will be shut up in an asylum or prison. It is a serious defect of the school system not yet to have provided special classes everywhere for children who are sane but difficult: for this is the sole hope of saving such a child if he is educable at all. (The doctors who examined E. abstained from any definite prognosis, and it was the duty of the teachers to try every known means before giving him up.)

As we have seen, Adlerian psychology recognizes no essential difference between a normal child and a difficult one, but it distinguishes the normal child from the abnormal (feeble-minded) by this criterion—that the feeble-minded lacks a directive line of life.

Dr. Birnbaum draws our attention to the importance of deciding whether it is the child's intellect (Verstand) or its reason (Vernunft) which is defective. He distinguishes:

The *normal*, whose intellect and reason are both sound.

The *a-social, neurotic* or *criminal*, whose reason is defective.

The *feeble-minded*, whose intellect is deficient.

There is only a difference of degree between the normal child and the difficult child whose reason (= social under-standing) is inadequately developed. The difficult child has sufficient intellect at its disposal, for its activity is appropriate to the ends it is trying to attain. It is enough to correct the fundamental error which makes it choose these ends on the negative side of life. The task of education is to prevent the difficult child from becoming an a-social being, a neurotic or a criminal. In these border-line cases, the school plays a part that is decisive for the whole of their future.

The course of the collective conversations illustrates very clearly how children make progress towards abstract thinking. The questions they discuss grow more and more general in character as the children's outlook widens to a more and more extensive horizon. At first it is predominantly points of order that arouse discussion, for it is the deepening of the notion of discipline that is the starting point for that long interior travail which leads from anarchy to autonomy. Later on come such questions as legible writing, the combative instinct, and religion, until one day there awakens, in the already ripening minds of the children, a sense of the illimitable indebtedness and duty of the individual to the community.

Other questions recur regularly; that of economizing, for instance, which renews its urgency every year in view of the school excursion. Thus when the time comes for leaving school, these children will have worked out a kind of practical philosophy, inspired by the principles of the Adlerian psychology.

Dr. Adler was once present at the last collective conversation of a class that was on the point of leaving school. The discussion turned upon the meaning of life, and the children arrived of themselves at this most characteristic Adlerian conclusion: the meaning of life is to make a contribution to the community. Dr. Adler was so surprised and moved at this that he felt unable to add a word.

According to Dr. Spiel, one would have to observe, in particular, children in the final year of their schooling in order to discover the best educators of to-morrow. For in the course of their collective discussions one can see, in some of them, that mysterious tact which enables one mind to enter into the minds of its companions. That faculty seems indeed indispensable to the fruitful practice of Adlerian method. Though all else may be acquired by will and application, this may well be innate, and should indicate, for the children who possess it, success in the educational calling. For in this, as in other things, the mere copyist can easily misapply all that is most ingenious and productive in the method. The experimental school alone is likely to furnish the masters who will be able to carry the Adlerian method on into the future.

CHAPTER FOUR

The Medico-Pedagogic Councils

A. GENERAL CONSIDERATIONS

Their necessity

THE first of these councils based on the psychology of Adler dates back to the year 1920. At that time the consequences of the world war were at their worst, and despite the admirable organization of Vienna, its childhood-protection service was quite inadequate to cope with the predicament of families and young people. Moral disintegration was progressive, and the number of young delinquents was growing from day to day. The need for immediate measures was imperative, and was felt as much in the educational as in the social sphere.

Such were the conditions in which Dr. Adler set up his first consultative groups. And as he had realized that the erroneous conduct of a child is always traceable to defective education, he created the councils as much for parents as for children. Far from being occupied only with difficult or ailing children, these councils intervened most successfully at the moment when the pedagogic methods of parents or teachers had proved ineffectual.

Their organization

At the beginning, these consultations were frequented only by teachers bringing difficult children with them, and seeking initiation into the Adlerian methods. (Lehrberatungsstellen.)

But the growing interest of the parents soon made it

necessary to find a place where they too could come to obtain advice about the educational procedures that they should adopt for their children (Erziehungsberatungsstellen). It was not long before such consultations constituted a living relation between the parents, the school and the doctors, and they have always been presided over by a consultant who had made the ideas of Adler his own.

All the consultations are free of charge. Each child becomes the subject of a dossier, in which is recorded all that can be learnt about it from its parents and its teachers, as well as all the conversations that have been held with it. The councils sit once or twice a week, usually about five or six o'clock in the evening, when the parents can more easily find time to accompany their child, and when the child also will be out of school. The success of these councils became so considerable that every district of the city wished to have one. They already numbered as many as twenty-six in 1929.

In most cases it is the schools who request a psychologist and a doctor, versed in Adlerian theory, to devote their services to this work on one or two evenings every week.

Their procedure

At the start of each school year, the masters are informed by circular of the existence, the place and times of the consultations. When the masters wish to refer a child to them, they have first to ask the permission of the parents, for these councils have no official or obligatory status. Whenever he can, the master attends them at the same time as the parents and the child in order that the collaboration of the educators may be as complete as possible. He will have previously notified the psychologist and the doctor, in the absence of the parents and the child, about the school record of the latter, its state of health and its behaviour in class, its difficulties and—so far as he knows it—about its family situation. In detail, the organization and the functioning of the councils vary considerably from district to district and according to the persons who conduct them. The majority of the councils are held in one of the school rooms. The consultant, his assistant (who records the minutes), the doctor, the parents and/or the child sit at the master's table and any others occupy the class-room desks. But of course one must not ascribe too much importance to these merely external factors which are frequently modified by circumstances.

It is not uncommon for the discussion of a case to take place before several masters from other schools, educators and others engaged in child-protection, who wish to profit by the experience. It is only later that the parents and the child are introduced. Some consultants like them to be present at the same time, to avoid arousing any mistrust, while others prefer to interrogate them separately so that each can speak out and unburden his or her mind as freely as they feel they need. Even here the method varies: some always wish to speak first with the parents, to avert any possible shock to whatever feelings of parental authority and prestige they may have; others on the contrary like to begin with the child in order to get an impression devoid of preconceived ideas. Dr. Adler himself receives the mother first and the child afterwards.

Numerous minor differences are noticeable to anyone making a round of these councils inspired by the Adlerian psychology. Those who direct them are fully aware of it when they depart from Adler's own 'model' consultative method, but each of them justifies in his own way the variation that he adopts.

When they have spoken with the parents and the child,

a second discussion is often held, at which the teacher most occupied with the child is enabled to brief himself to the best advantage on his pupil's behalf.

In these days, propitious family environments are certainly exceptional, so that the major responsibility for education now devolves upon the school. Hence the extreme importance of action upon the educators, upon whom the success of the child's re-education will generally depend.

Not infrequently parents take the initiative in presenting themselves with their child to a council, having heard of its work through some acquaintances or at a lecture. One also finds guardians of children bringing their charges for advice.

The diagnosis invariably commences with the medical report, in order to be sure that the child in question is not incapable of doing better. But the number of feeble-minded is happily very small. On the other hand it commonly happens, as we have seen, that a child believed to suffer from a mental disease proves after all to be only excessively discouraged. If so, a change of masters and a new attitude on the part of the parents may work miracles. It is noteworthy that the councils only rarely resort to tests in estimating the degree of a child's development. They rely chiefly upon educational inquiries and brief, frank interviews.

Although he well knows that symptoms are but the indications of an attitude that is erroneous as a whole, the psychologist never fails to question the parents about the faults of which they complain. Many of them do not realize that it is the whole attitude of the child that interests the psychologist. The latter has therefore to proceed by progressively widening the scope of the conversation until he has obtained all the information that may be important. In most instances the parents are able to recall the precise moment at which they began to notice the behaviour of which they complain; and this nearly always coincides with some new situation to which the child was unable to adapt itself. This may have been the birth of a little brother or sister, the entry into kindergarten or into school, a change of master, or removal to another town, an excessive masturbation, or again it may have been a great fright (caused by a large dog, for example).

When a child in need of re-education is found to be in an extremely unfavourable environment, its removal is obligatory.

It is for the observation of such cases that one feels the need of a special *home* (such as that of the city of Vienna which we have described elsewhere) administered upon Adlerian principles. Unhappily no such institution yet exists, although one may consider as an attempt in that direction the 'Nachmittagshort' of Fräulein Friedmann, where the children spend the afternoons at their lessons and can remain to play until seven o'clock under the supervision of an expert observer. In such a home for observation, one could decide what should be done with a child who has to be taken away from its family, and its re-education could be undertaken in such a way that it would be subsequently returned to its family without danger of a relapse into its morbid condition. At the same time, one would endeavour to influence the parents so that they would not renew their previous errors. Such a child would, of course, need to be treated with special care upon its return to the school, until it had become re-established in its environment.

After the first visit to a council, a child may come again, alone or accompanied by its parents, as the case requires. It should be encouraged by some little positive successes of which it can speak to the psychologist, who thereby begins to exercise a control based upon mutual confidence. If it is a matter of rendering the child more independent it will be asked, according to circumstances, to dress itself without aid, or to eat politely and without fuss, to do its duties by itself, to assist its mother by helping its brothers and sisters, to help its schoolfellows, to make a friend, etc. . . .

In specially refractory cases, the council may seek a lay assistant, versed in the psychology of Adler, who looks after the child some hours every day. In this service very real sacrifices are made by persons who love children more than themselves, since there can never be any question of remuneration from such impoverished clients.

It can never be over-emphasized that the essential task of the doctor, psychologist and teacher in conducting these councils, is to grasp as quickly as they can the 'plan of life' pursued by whoever comes to them for aid. Nor is it only a matter of understanding this; they must also know how to explain it to the child, to demonstrate what is wrong in its conduct. The consultant therefore needs not only to have an extensive knowledge of psychology at his disposal; he must also be skilled in the art of putting his science into practice.

Their objective

At bottom these consultations are an attempt to do what neither the family nor the kindergarten have succeeded in doing (and in which the school of itself cannot well succeed): to give the child something it ought to have had from its mother. The children presented to the councils are discouraged beings, suffering from lack of confidence in themselves and in those around them. Their deficient feeling for community has made them incapable of a positive attitude. The pedagogue has therefore to try, first and foremost, to win the child's confidence, the indispensable preliminary to any radical improvement.

What the child needs is to acquire the feeling that its adviser is a man upon whom it can count at all times, in no matter what situation; a friend who wants to get it out of a scrape. This first stage safely passed, the educator will begin to detach the child from him personally, for the best deed that the little one could ever do would have no objective value if it were done only to please him. The educator now seeks little by little to re-orientate the child towards the society in which it will have to live, trying to render the adaptation as little painful as possible. However weak and discouraged an individual may seem to be, one can always discover a little flame of social courage still burning dimly somewhere within him.

We have already insisted so much upon the importance of the parents' attitude that there is no need to repeat that this work ought never to be limited to the child alone. Its reformation depends so largely upon the understanding of the parents that the pedagogue can never do too much to win their confidence. What is needed is to make them understand, at the same time as the child, both the internal and external factors which have provoked a deviation of behaviour in the absence of an adequate educational method. In certain cases, the consultant may even be able to see that he would have acted in the same way if he had been placed in the same circumstances. Just so far as the parents and the child recognize their previous error, they will acquire a firmer and more courageous attitude. The burden upon the present is invariably some need to liquidate the past.

Most of the consultations are held in public. This is the aspect of them most often singled out for attack; it is supposed that such publicity must hamper both parents and children; that they must often be ill at ease in the presence of up to twenty persons. Yet this method of procedure actually presents more advantage than inconvenience in a great many cases. It often has a happy effect upon the child, who is reassured by the sympathy of a number of persons so much interested in its welfare. This may also give the child a feeling that its difficulties are those of many others and that it is natural enough to come and consult competent persons about such things. It no longer feels alone with its troubles; it is not ashamed of itself, nor are its parents. It goes to the council as one goes to the dentist when suffering from a decayed tooth. And there, perhaps for the first time, it finds itself talking to an adult who has divested himself of all that 'authority' so willingly assumed by persons who feel incapable of creating mutual confidence between themselves and children. For the first time, perhaps, the child feels it is understood and treated with respect by some 'grown-ups'. It then sees the auditors less as judges than as friends who understand and want to come to its assistance.

When the public character of the councils is used in this way, it certainly assists towards the development of the child's sociability.

The ideal pursued by those who give these consultations is the formation of independent personalities, apt for co-operation; healthy and upright individuals capable of overcoming all their difficulties. They advise each one who consults them how to liquidate his failures and find the courage to make a new attempt. But they endeavour, at the same time, to infuse with their own spirit as many other teachers and lovers of children as they can. It is a fact that no one comes away from one of these consultations without having profited by it directly or indirectly. We must add, however, that admission to a session is suspended, if the parents formally object to publicity or if a child obstinately declines to speak in the presence of others. And some of the medical psychologists will only hold sessions in their own consulting-rooms, in the presence of not more than three others.

SUMMARY

The psychologist must endeavour to grasp as swiftly and also as completely as possible, the plan of life formed by an individual, and then ask himself how he can best win his confidence. Then he will try to enable the individual to recognize the inanity of the aim which has been determining his behaviour. Step by step, as a child regains confidence in its own ability, the psychologist will also re-orientate it towards society, and enable it to recover, little by little, its rightful place in the bosom of the community.

All these stages have to be successfully negotiated if an educator does not want to leave his task half-done but is truly seeking to render the individual in his charge able to educate himself in the future. If he attempts a short cut, he will only get an illusory success. We now know well enough that the Adlerian does not go out of his way to eliminate this or that troublesome symptom. He seeks rather to seize its meaning in relation to the personality as a whole, in order to open the way to a radical transformation of the style of life. His aim is to reveal a new goal in harmony with the requirements of communal living.

B. TYPES OF CHILDREN

Before trying broadly to classify the types of children who show marked difficulties in the course of their development, it must be said that they are almost all characterized by lack of communal feeling.

Dr. Adler divides them into three groups of which we have said something already on pages 42 and 43.

(1) Spoilt children (verzärtelte Kinder).

(2) Hated children (gehasste Kinder).

(3) Children with organic inferiorities (organminder-wertige Kinder).

The spoilt children do not succeed in adapting to a new situation because an over-anxious mother, misunderstanding her duties, has done her utmost to clear every obstacle from their path. Brought up 'in cottonwool', such children become incapable of accomplishing the simplest thing when left to themselves, and at the same time expect praise and admiration for their every gesture. What is to be wondered at if a child of this character is discouraged when it enters school? No one has hitherto dared ask it to perform a service, still less required it to make the smallest effort; and here it is, suddenly plunged into surroundings where its position is in no way distinguished from that of others, in which it can no longer feel the mother's protective hand! Never having had to win anyone's confidence, not knowing in the least how to behave in order to attract the friendship of its schoolfellows, it will soon be exhibiting symptoms tending to prove to its family that it has no use for school and had better be withdrawn from it. It may be a long performance, every morning, to make such a child get up. Often it will go so far as to be sick, thus engrossing the mother's attention and gaining the right to miss an hour, if not a whole morning, at school.

One must never neglect to inform oneself about what we have called the 'family constellation' of a child. More often than not, in these days, one finds one is dealing with an only child. This situation, which used to be exceptional, is becoming almost the rule; we have seen classes of which a good half were 'only' children. This is a development that renders the kindergarten a still more imperative necessity, for it enables such children to have the experience, often wholly lacking at home, of a real community.

Here is a rebellious child who refuses to eat; who makes endless scenes at the family table every day. The parents' most efficacious response to this is the passive one, an apparently total disregard of the matter. If the child really doesn't want to eat, it is better it should not do so, for nourishment taken against its will cannot do it much good. Leave it then to sulk behind its plate till the meal is over! One may be sure that after one or two fruitless demonstrations it will again take to its food . . . that is, as soon as the child realizes that its parents do not react as they used to, and are not worrying themselves about its abstinence. Thenceforth the child will eat according to appetite and custom without attaching extraneous value to the act. It of course depends upon the age and the understanding of the child whether one can usefully explain to it, in direct terms, what it is trying to gain by its obstinacy—in this case by not wanting to eat—or whether it is best to proceed indirectly. One may, for instance, tell the child a story about a little rebel who behaved in a somewhat similar fashion, and go on to narrate how this person learnt to overcome all his difficulties. This tactic is often enough successful. In the case of a child who is already set upon a certain profession, one can often make effective use of the imagination in relation to its future career; one can show it how the success to which it aspires depends upon its growing up in harmony with society.

C. MISTAKES THAT ADVISERS MAY MAKE

1. *Vanity and over-assurance caused by success*

It goes without saying that the success of the consultations depends also upon the consultant, and that errors on his part may provoke a set-back. One consultant may readily succeed with a case which another could bring to no conclusion. Certain psychologists who have a marvellous competence in all the necessary knowledge, and understand clearly what is wrong with their patient's plan of life, are nevertheless unable to direct him into the right way for lack of sufficient tact or adequate authority.

As we have already had occasion to remark, the psychologist needs constantly to maintain as objective an attitude as possible towards those under his treatment. If he acquires a subjective interest in his patient's cure it will almost inevitably miscarry. The consultant himself needs to act always in view of the community. He has to take good care that no success flatters his vanity, and above all he must never give any advice whatever from personal interest or ambition, i.e., he must never be trying to make a name for himself by the number of successes he can add to his credit. This is a snare which too many beginners do not know how to avoid. The more convinced he is of the principles he professes, the more objective a psychologist needs to be about his manner of practising them. His firmness and tranquillity will then always have a beneficent influence upon those who come to him for help.

2. *The danger of stopping half-way*

Another danger lurks in what Freud calls the 'transference'. An educator may easily manage to do duty for the mother and establish between himself and the child a relationship that gives it confidence. He sometimes forgets that he has to discharge the second duty of motherhood, to sever the attachment he has created and direct the child's interest towards society. If he does not go on to this second phase, such success as he has will be based only upon the sympathy he inspires in the child, who will not recognize in its inner consciousness that to act in such and such ways is a duty it owes itself. Then the whole question is merely postponed to another day, when perhaps the child's interest in the educator weakens, or when the latter has dismissed it as cured. In that case the educator has indeed stopped half-way, not having known how to give the child the magic key of self-education.

3. *Change of home is not lightly to be prescribed*

Other educators too readily wish to alter unfavourable family circumstances. They straightway prescribe a change of environment, which is indeed indicated in very many cases. Dr. Adler however recommends that everything else should be tried before taking a child out of its natural setting. For what he wants is precisely that children should learn how to live in their own circumstances, coping with all the difficulties that these present to them, in which their characters may be shaped and strengthened.

4. *The disappearance of symptoms is not enough*

The educator needs also to resist the temptation to try to satisfy the parents too quickly, when this may be to the detriment of the child. The disappearance of a troublesome symptom means nothing of itself; as we know, the real cure is of something much deeper. An educator has to act upon the inner consciousness of the child; otherwise his influence will prove itself superficial and transient. To this end he will try to identify himself with a child he wants to re-educate. That is the best way to find the correct attitude, neither too formal nor too familiar; it also enables him to proceed with the utmost objectivity, bearing in mind however that his own subjectivity cannot be wholly eliminated; indeed, the irreducible element of subjectivity is what distinguishes the true pedagogue, and makes him able to feel and to follow like an artist the innumerable little variations of meaning which even the most apparently similar symptoms never cease to present.

We must here raise a point of difficulty that is inherent not only in these councils inspired by Adler's psychology, but in advisory methods in general. Being unable to constrain anybody in any way whatever, their function being purely advisory, the official character of such councils implies the *impossibility of any control*. For example, one hardly ever knows to what extent the mothers put into practice the recommendations so freely made to them; one can only go by what they or their children say. It is true that, when a re-education is already advanced, one can estimate the parents' collaboration by results. But the road to perdition is paved with good intentions. It is a long road from the consultation to the house; good intentions have time to dwindle on the way, and perhaps vanish altogether when exposed to the habitual atmosphere of home.

One can hardly imagine how delicately the psychologist has to proceed, to bring a re-education to success without exhausting the patience of the parents. In this capital city the distances are great, the tramways tiresome. Can we wonder if some parents cease to attend the council or, what is worse, are overheard making disagreeable remarks? They came at first because they were complaining of their child's misbehaviour and thought they would find a personal ally in the psychologist; and here he is, actually taking the child's part in some respects, even reproaching them for their ideas about its upbringing!

Clearly, re-education conducted without controls is likely to be made longer. At the beginning things go well enough, provided one does not shock the parents by some clumsiness. But later on, one may well go on telling them, in every possible tone of voice, that these cases take time to cure: still, they break off the treatment, and one sees them no more, never knowing exactly why. Generally they have found the change they were expecting too long in coming: their child has given some fresh trouble despite the consultations . . . so these must be worthless and the parents decide to go back to the 'firm method', which they now think they ought never to have abandoned . . . they blame themselves only for not having been severe enough before. Or they satisfy themselves with the oft-repeated argument: 'It is a waste of time trying to reform such a child as this'. In some cases these parents come back again after a few months, having applied in vain every method that their untrained reason could suggest to them, and in despair of understanding the case they want the council to have one more try before they leave things to take their course. If the psychologist is very clever, if he has tact enough to inspire new confidence in parents thus returning to him full of doubt and mistrust, he may yet perhaps manage to score a success despite an initial failure.

Thus it is not possible as yet to draw up any statistics about the councils' successes. Their records are at once too summary (since parents and children attend too irregularly) and too incomplete (one cannot always tell whether those who have ceased to attend did so because they think all is well now or for the opposite reason). Parents rarely seem to think it worth while to inform the psychologist of their reasons for ceasing to present themselves.

In default of a statistical record, the best way to inform ourselves about the variety of cases treated at the councils would be, we should think, an inquiry into all the difficulties that arise in the course of a child's education. We should then see that there are difficulties characteristic of each age-group, precipitated in the first place by external circumstances, such as the entry into school. Certain difficulties, of course, are also to be found at any age vary-ing with the attitudes assumed by the parents.

D. DESCRIPTION AND EXPLANATION OF CASES PRESENTED TO THE COUNCILS

It is not easy to decide upon any scheme of classification; children are brought to the councils for such a vast variety of reasons. We know, too, that the psychologist looks beyond these reasons. Whether a mother brings her little girl because she is continually disobedient, or because she will not go to school, makes scenes at table or, again, because she wets her bed—he will regard the external sign only as a clue for the discovery of the goal at which the child is aiming. Usually, as we have seen, the child is only trying to draw the attention of the parents to itself. On the other hand the family's situation, or its economic con-dition (e.g. unemployment) may exert an influence so decisive that these factors cannot be omitted in a classification.

However, we will base our remarks upon the age of the child, and consider the difficulties that are most commonly related to it. Any classification must inevitably be more or less arbitrary, for life never exactly repeats itself: but some groupings appear to be necessary in order to grasp the various problems that come before the councils.

The babies

Education necessarily begins from the child's birth, and if well conducted strengthens its character for the rest of its life. With quite small babies, the difficulties encountered are almost always those of feeding and sleeping; it is these that arouse the earliest reactions, often misunderstood by the adults in charge; in which case the baby is in danger of becoming a nervous child and, later on, an adult neuropath. Adler's ideas are no less valuable in the care of those that are called 'naughty' babies because they exasperate parents and others by continual crying. Neither type is at all rare, but it is not often that a mother presents a council with difficulties of either kind. She usually prefers to go for advice to a parents' union (Elternverein) or a mothers' union (Mütterverein) where she has every freedom to raise questions and even to play an active part, perhaps with some pride, in discussing whatever questions may be worrying her.

At two or three years of age, one can already make useful appeal to a child's understanding, but that is obviously impossible with a nursling, which has of necessity to be left exclusively to its mother. The important thing is that she should be helped to realize her two essential duties and how best to fulfil them in the existing circumstances. The baby's behaviour will follow from her attitude towards it. Will she be able to ensure for it that first and indispensable feeling of confidence in life? And will she know how to detach it from herself at the right time, transferring its attention to the other members of the family, especially the father, whose function we have already noted?

We may seem to be attributing exaggerated importance to the earliest influences a child is subjected to. But we have been convinced by experience, in all the difficult cases we have encountered, that no substantial alteration can take place unless one succeeds in fulfilling the primary duty to the child which its mother has not discharged. That is why an adult neurotic or criminal cannot get back into the straight way until and unless his re-educator succeeds in giving him these two fundamental experiences—of confidence in himself and others, and then of the existence of the human community to which we all belong, and to which each individual contributes by every one of his actions.

The youngest child ever brought before the councils during our six months' observation of them was two and a half years old. She was an example of *the child tyrannizing over its parents*. Hardly had the mother entered the council when, in the presence of her little girl (from whom, as we shall see, she could not separate herself for a single moment) she began to complain of her child's exaggerated attachment. It would never consent to leave her. Every night, after two or three hours' sleep, it would suddenly awaken and cry until the mother took it into her bed. The mother having declined any longer to 'obey' in this manner, the child had immediately resorted to another device. She began again to wet her bed, a thing which had not happened since she was one year old. In the daytime the mother could not leave the little one alone for any length of time but she would alarm the neighbours by her weeping and screaming. To avoid such scenes, the mother felt obliged to take her little daughter with her wherever she went. We learned that the father was a designer of advertisements for a cinema; he was excessively occupied, and had neither the time nor the inclination to pay much attention to his daughter, to whom he said nothing beyond a perfunctory greeting when he came home. The mother, a woman of thirty-seven, had been an actress before her marriage, and was now dissatisfied with merely domestic and maternal duties; moreover, she herself suffered from her husband's over-work, which made him come home late every evening, showing no interest in anything but to get to sleep as quickly as possible. To add that the daughter was the only child is almost needless; a child accustomed to share everything, including the mother, with brothers and sisters would never have been able to tyrannize over its mother to the point of subjecting her wholly to its will.

From the attitude of the mother at this consultation we

could easily discern the grievance that she was tacitly directing against her husband: she, who had once been surrounded by admirers, was now wounded by his indifference. The first advice given to her was to take her little girl immediately to a Montessorian kindergarten— the only one which admitted children less than three years old; for her own nervous condition prevented her from behaving as the child needed that she should. A discouraged and deprived person, troubled to the depths of her being, cannot know, even though she has the best of intentions, how to give a child the confidence it so much needs; for her own condition will never wholly escape the sensitive apprehension of the child. To inspire confidence one must have it.

Not without difficulty, the father was prevailed upon to attend the council on one occasion. In the course of an intimate conversation, the doctor found he had to do with a case of impotence. We thus understand more and more of the difficulty this child must have to find its equilibrium in surroundings so full of bitterness. The mother resents the father's weakness, and the father suffers in turn from the injustice of his wife, who reproaches him with an 'illness' for which he is far from feeling responsible. The child suffers from the mistrust inherent in such a state of things, and tries to compensate for its sense of vital insecurity by contriving the closest possible relationship between herself and the mother. Never having played with another child, the little girl is naturally very timid and fearful.

But the link it creates with the mother is in no way positive or intimate. Its nature is, so to speak, purely negative, consisting solely in the fear of its being broken. This means that nothing productive can come of it. A child who has need of all its little strength to *prevent* something from happening, has no resources left for normal development.

One therefore endeavours to influence the mother, to make her understand that her duty for the moment is to oppose her child as little as possible, leaving it the utmost liberty to live by the ideas suggested to it by the kindergarten or at the consultations, and even encouraging it to activity. Meanwhile the doctor will treat the father for his infirmity.

During the whole period of re-education, one cannot too constantly advise the parents to treat each other with all possible indulgence, since they both feel they are animated by the same desire to free themselves from a situation they regard as intolerable. The consultant, for his part, is more hopeful when a situation becomes insupportable, for the genuine will to a radical cure can only arise from the suffering that such a predicament causes. One may observe, by the way, that this is so for our bodily organism; only when pain tells us that something is not functioning as it should, do we decide to take care of ourselves.

In a case such as we have just outlined, a great step has already been taken when the consultant has managed to dispel the bitterness that was poisoning the relations between the two parents. It will not be long before mutual confidence is reborn—or rather born, for they have never really experienced that benign condition.

The reformation of a whole family requires a long and indeed painful labour, for it is only possible through the intimate collaboration between them all. The parents and the child have to present themselves regularly at the council once or twice a week till an effective contact is established between all concerned. Moreover, particular advice has to be given to the kindergarten mistress in charge of the re-education of the child. The child itself, by means of the little services it is being induced to render to schoolfellows, will gradually grow sociable; and by the time it has to go to school, it will have become a courageous little person and able to adapt itself properly to any new situation.

Our conclusion is that parents cannot too soon resort to the councils with their children whenever they see them in difficulties of any importance. The personal life of the parents themselves may derive unexpected benefit from this. 'By a curious reversal of rôles, the child may indeed become the educator of its parents!' (Adler.)

The child attending kindergarten

Little H., a girl of five, is brought before a council because of her continual disobedience. She presents an example of *the spoiled child demanding its 'rights'*. Every day this little thing makes scenes which come to a climax at meal-times, when she cannot be made to eat anything without promptly vomiting.

—We have tried everything, gentleness as well as firmness. Nothing does any good. Whatever can we do with her?

And the parents go on to tell us all the difficulties they have to make her get up in the mornings.

We learn from the doctor that the little hussy enjoys quite good health. When she was on holiday at a children's camp, she was so far from refusing to eat that she was soon known as a 'hearty eater' and envied for it. However, as soon as those around her became accustomed to this characteristic and paid no more attention to it, the little girl again began to refuse to eat. Thus she attained the same end in a new way, again becoming a centre of attention. But she went so far that they had to ask her mother to come and take her away, for no one could prevail on her to eat anything at all.

We will record a part of the conversation that ensued at the first consultation.

(*M.* = mother,   *C.* = consultant,   *H.* = the child.)

M. Before coming here, H. asked me if they would give her anything to eat here too.

C. You see the enormous importance she attaches to anything to do with food. She understands its immense importance in all our lives and is availing herself of this to draw your attention to her. This is a child who does not yet dare to go far from its parents: she is trying to keep herself, as long as possible, as a baby, whose mother lives almost entirely for it.

M. What annoys me most of all is that she wants to get up at six o'clock on Sunday, the one day on which we can sleep a little longer, and yet it is hard enough to get her up at half-past seven on weekdays, in time to go to her kindergarten.

C. The little one is assuming every morning an attitude of opposition, of obstinacy. So we had better—at least at the beginning—try to make things a little more attractive for her. We won't say anything to her, if you please, about her eating or not eating. If we do she will immediately suppose that that is the point of most importance to us, and she will only renew her demonstrations at home. May we ask you, then, to keep to yourself what we have just said?

As soon as the mother has left the room the child enters it with very firm steps. She looks very wide awake and active.

C. Well, you do know how to come into a room and sit on a chair, just like a big person! Do you also know how to get up in the mornings?

H. No.

C. Oh, well, you will soon learn. When mother calls you to-morrow morning, you will get up at once, and tell her that from now on you want to dress yourself every morning just as grown-up people do.

H. Yes.

The mother comes again several times, without any improvement to report. She is rather unresponsive to the advice given her; she too easily loses patience and again resorts to whipping the little girl. However, one has at all costs to avoid anything that might discourage her altogether and keep her away from the council. When the psychologist gently reproaches her, reminding her that last time she herself admitted that the 'firm method' led nowhere, she retorts that she is only sorry she didn't adopt it sooner, for, she says, the little girl at least obeys at the moment when she is punished. It is most difficult to get her to see that there is no point in an artificial and temporary 'cure', that by such means she is in danger of making the child a little rebel.

From a conversation between the psychologist and the little girl, one can easily understand how she has come to imagine her fellow beings. She is one of those who are never satisfied unless they have some extraordinary part to play, and think they have a right to everything without giving anything in return.

C. Do you like playing with your schoolfellows?

H. Yes.

C. Do you get on well with them?

H. No, not at all, they're always slapping me.

C. Why do they do that?

H. Because they want to.

C. Perhaps you haven't been kind to them.

H. Oh yes, I'm always kind.

C. Do you think it's possible for one child always to be good and the others always naughty?

H. Yes, I'm always good, and they're always naughty.

C. Do you say 'good morning' nicely to them every day when you come into the class-room?

H. No, I never say good morning.

C. Why is that?

H. I don't want to.

C. But you see, the other children don't know that you're not saying good morning because you don't want to. They only think you're sulky if you never greet them. Come now, go out quickly, and see if you can say good morning when you come in again. Run along!

The child goes out and, coming back again, holds out her hand very politely to the persons seated near the door.

C. There, you knew how to say good morning just like a grown-up person! Will you try to do the same to-morrow morning at kindergarten?

H. Yes.

C. And if another child asks you to do something for her, you will, won't you? For you have to show them that you like them, they don't know it yet.

In this case, the mother proved so refractory to the psychologist's advice that he had ultimately to rely upon the favourable factor of the kindergarten, laying upon its young mistress the tasks that were properly incumbent upon the mother. As soon as the feeling for community began to develop in the child it was easier to induce the mother to do her own part towards the liberation and independence of this lively little girl, who only needed to be led in the right way. The mother did not change her ways until she could see for herself the results of an education which kept to the golden mean between excessive severity and exaggerated gentleness. There were some set-backs, but that is always

132

to be expected. And in the end the child became very sociable, and well able to co-operate.

Over-ambitious upbringing

A little girl M., five years old, is brought by her father because she is extremely *nervous*, and wets her bed nearly every night.

The father is out of work. And, being extremely ambitious, he suffers especially from the fact that it is his wife who has to keep them by work as a seamstress. He is preyed upon almost continually by insomnia. These circumstances obviously exert an unfavourable influence upon the development of little M. Since the mother can give her but a very little time each day, the parental functions have to be reversed, and the father has the more to do with her. But, living in a state of almost constant depression, he cannot give his child a proper upbringing. He has to resort to strong measures, and he goes as far as to stay beside the little girl, cane in hand, for the whole of a meal-time! After that, is it so surprising if the child exhibits symptoms of fear and insecurity or if she wets her bed?

Here, since it is needful above all to modify the father's regrettable way of living, one first of all puts it to him that it is excessive 'respect' for her father (not to say her terrible fear of him) which is making the little girl so timid. Knowing almost nothing of the mother's love (her mamma comes home late at night) which she so badly needs, she tries to secure some of it at night, if only by a stratagem of despair. She thus proceeds to wet the bed, which she never did when she was quite tiny and was boarded out with her grandparents.

To encourage the father is difficult. One can imagine what a tragedy it is, for such an ambitious man to find himself facing a void day after day, after having toiled for fifteen years in hopes of attaining a good position. At first he did all he could think of to find another situation, but no kind of work was offered him. Then, from day to day his energies declined, and now we have to do with a man who is old at forty, who is expecting no more from life and has abandoned hope. The last traces of his former activity appear in his attitude to his daughter. But even the ambition that he cherishes for her future lacks any consistency, for he can really see no meaning in life since it has deprived him of his right to work.

To find an occupation for this unhappy father was impossible. One could but endeavour, not without some measure of success, to re-awaken his faith in a better future. The little one, in spite of her tender years, was accessible to our explanations. She could understand her father's great sadness, and there was something tragic in seeing such misery reflected in the soul of a child. But we could not spare her the ordeal because she was beginning to doubt her father's love, and on that point she had to be reassured.

A spark of hope revived in the heart of the father on the day when the child had not wetted its bed. Then after some weeks of improvement, we saw no more of him. We can but hope it was because psychological help was no longer needed, and that his re-employment left him no time to come again.

In these days unemployment has become an agonizing problem. Those who are fortunate enough to have work have too much of it, for which they and their families suffer. But the fate of the unemployed is worse, for besides the bitterness of their privation, they have all too much time for those innumerable family complications which give rise to interminable dissensions. Promiscuous housing in exiguous quarters, under-nourishment, almost incessant mutual reproaches—all these things make up a bitter and stifling atmosphere.

When one has seen, vegetating in one hovel, families of five, six and even seven persons, one is never again astonished by their delinquencies. We may almost congratulate ourselves that these are not more common than they are.

Schoolchildren up to fourteen years old

The majority of the children brought before the councils are schoolchildren between six and fourteen years of age. Entry into school signifies for every child the beginning of a new life. It marks the first real contact with society and the child's social feeling is put to a searching test. Above all is this so for one who has not been through the kindergarten, especially if, in addition, it is an 'only' child.

We have seen that the attitude the child assumes towards its new surroundings depends mainly upon what its mother has been able to do for it. Has she given it its first, indispensable experience of confidence? Has she then detached it sufficiently from herself to orientate it, through the father's mediation, towards the community? When the mother, for one reason or another, proves unequal to her task, the kindergarten often succeeds in supplying this important deficiency before it has had time to entail serious consequences.

There is a double burden on a child's shoulders from the moment it enters the school. On the one hand, it has to find its place by its own efforts in the new environment, neither to be overcome by it nor to deviate from it in one way or another. On the other hand, it has to acquire, in a relatively short time, a certain amount of indispensable knowledge; to learn to read, write and calculate. The child who is ill-prepared for the common life thus finds itself placed between two tasks of which either would be enough to tax all its strength; a thorough change in its behaviour, and the acquisition of necessary knowledge.

It is no wonder if, from then on, many children fall by the way—if they 'deviate' and begin to exhibit troublesome symptoms which they had never shown before. That was simply because they had no need, for everything seemed to go along smoothly by itself (for which read 'by the mother'). From the first school day the child that is unprepared for common life feels itself inferior; and it will try to hide this feeling, or to make up for it in some direction outside the community.

We have already said that no classification of the cases treated by a council can be based upon the symptoms for which they are brought to its notice, and we have seen why.

At school, certain children have no difficulties except in learning. Their attitudes towards their school-mates leave nothing to be desired; their *scholarship* alone is in question. There are others, sometimes among the best for their scholarship, who cannot manage to adapt their behaviour to their new surroundings. In most cases, however, children manifest some difficulties both in scholarship and in behaviour, which is natural since the two aspects are closely related. There is often indeed a vicious circle: bad work at lessons provokes bad behaviour, because the child tries to procure somewhere else a satisfaction he has failed to find in his school work. He may then easily become unruly, may lie or pilfer, or in the worst case grow aggressive. By tics or grimaces he will capture the attention if he cannot win the admiration of his comrades. And this ill-behaviour will in turn prevent his following the lessons till the distance separating him from the class may widen into a gulf. Then the child 'contracts out' altogether, either definitely withdraws behind his discouragement and acts the part of the 'stupid' or apathetic child or else becomes so savage that the least approach by his master or any schoolfellow becomes impossible. He will become a child of the type that one sees sitting apathetically on the lowest forms or, during recreations, munching his piece of bread alone in a corner.

We will now tabulate the difficulties that most often recur, first reminding our readers that the children presented before the councils are hardly ever above the age of fourteen.

I. DIFFICULTIES ARISING AT HOME

Relating to behaviour: possible symptoms

Exasperating disobedience ⎫
Intolerable unsociability ⎬ a-sociality—delinquency
Dangerous aggressiveness ⎭
Headaches ⎫
Stomach troubles, vomiting |
Tics (grimaces) ⎬ neurosis—psychopathy
Bad habits (e.g., enuresia) |
Excessive timidity: onanism ⎭

II. DIFFICULTIES ARISING IN SCHOOL

In relation to learning

A set-back in all subjects
A set-back in one subject
In arithmetic—calculative work generally
(often spoilt children)
In writing ⎫
In reading ⎬ (often awkward children)

Relating to behaviour: possible symptoms

Rebellious, obstreperous children, aggressive, untruthful,

pilfering; children who are timid, afraid, apathetic or 'model children'.

(The difficulties relating to work are very frequently involved with those due to behaviour.)

III. DIFFICULTIES ARISING OUT-OF-DOORS

In respect of behaviour: possible symptoms

Delinquency (theft, attacks upon passers-by).

From the presence of one or more of these symptoms the psychologist may locate the child's weak point, psychic or physical. But he will take this as no more than an introduction to the interior life of the child, never losing sight of the fact that manifest symptoms merely represent desperate efforts to compensate for a feeling of inferiority and to satisfy its will to power. For an Adlerian psychologist, all symptoms are equally grave, for all bear witness to an insufficient personal preparedness for independence and co-operation. It is this point of view that constitutes the chief originality of Adlerian practice, and affords the insight, luminous in its simplicity, that is so easily dismissed as 'banal' or 'over-simplified'. But whoever follows its application at first hand cannot fail to be impressed by the fruitfulness of a method which traces every error and perversity back to certain influences that were present, or others that were lacking, during early childhood. This conception has the merit of taking us back to origins, right back to the primary data. The knowledge it enables us to gain, of the most intimate and often unsuspected realities, not only enriches but changes one's own personality and, in consequence, one's attitude towards all children.

We will now turn to our records of a few cases. First of all, here is an instance of *the excessively jealous child* (Lehndorff-Krauss).

The child. Paul, twelve years old, delicate-looking and under weight.

Reason for seeking advice. Bed-wetting at night since the age of seven.

Family. The father is out of work. The mother takes great care of her children but spoils them too much, which has rendered them timid, especially Paul the eldest who is still treated like a baby. He has a sister of nine of whom he is terribly jealous, and he is easily angered.

School. The child is in the class appropriate to his age, but now, for the first time, is falling behind, his school work deteriorating, especially in arithmetic and German.

Profession. He would like to be a hairdresser, but cannot say what particularly attracts him to that occupation.

Earliest memories. Little Paul is afraid; afraid of everything, but especially of water, of fire, and of serpents (Freud). He remembers having cut his finger one day when he wanted to help his mother, and that he dropped the cup that he was putting in its place.

Dreams. Numerous, also about being frightened. The child dreams he is overcome by vertigo, or that he is falling down a mountain.

Interpretation of the case

This is a spoiled child who cannot grow out of the jealousy he feels about his little sister. Believing that she is preferred by the parents, he is trying to retain their attention by wetting his bed—i.e., by reproducing a situation experienced when he was a baby. It matters little to him that his parents scold him for this so long as they renew their attentions to him as they did when he was the only child. He can at least manage to concentrate their interest upon the question 'Has Paul wetted his bed?' and, as no reproaches or punishments can put a stop to this incontinence, the parents are brought to believe there must be some organic trouble and treat him with especial care. The child, then, has for the moment won the game, for his parents apply themselves to spoiling him as before. But this 'victory' entails a diminution of confidence, it is a hindrance to his independence and his development. His work at school consequently grows worse from week to week, till the day when the master asks the parents to take their child to the council, lest he should have to be put down into a lower class.

All this has come about simply because the mother did not know how to prepare the child for entry into communal living. Little Paul has quite naturally regarded his sister as his rival, and the idea of helping her in the capacity of elder brother has never entered his mind. The mother is at first extremely surprised when we demonstrate the relations between her son's jealousy, his bad habit and his unsatisfactory school work, but she soon arrives at a very good understanding.

Treatment. We undertake to evoke an admission of this relation from the boy himself. Appealing to his dignity, we then assure him that he is quite able to wake up when he needs to urinate. We emphasize the confidence we feel in him, in his desire to outgrow a habit so unsuitable at his age, and in his maturity which will enable him successfully to second our efforts. Then we advise him to do a little physical culture and swimming, to tone up his body and train him in physical and mental courage. Moreover, a mistress trained in Adlerian methods gives him lessons in arithmetic and German twice a week, to keep his re-education under supervision.

A rapid improvement is reported, and soon three weeks have gone by without another bed-wetting.

He has a *relapse* immediately after leaving his grandmother whom he greatly loves. We do not worry about this; it only shows us that his psychic fortitude is still insufficient to cope with an unwelcome situation. We explain this to him. The boy feels that he is becoming more and more grown-up, and aware that there is no need to resort to infantile measures in order to be assured of his parents' affection. After a few months he is so well re-established that of his own initiative he joins a band of scouts. Growing more sociable, he makes several friends and his performance of the daily 'good deed' required of each scout is quite heartfelt. His interest is now well redirected towards others, whereas he used to be afraid of them, and this has entirely transformed his attitude to his little sister. He is now proud of her and likes to feel himself her protector.

Overjoyed at all this, the mother came back several times to give thanks for the radical alteration not only in her son but in the whole family.

Owing to the absence of control over the majority of the cases, it would be a dubious matter to attempt any numerical record of the cures obtained by these consultations. Such statistics would vary a good deal according to the 'scientific conscience' of the consultant. Some of these are satisfied with an improvement reported at the moment when the child leaves off attending the council. Others never speak of a cure unless improvement has been maintained for some months; others again, not until the child has proved itself capable of courageously overcoming specific obstacles. There is no doubt that a child must have passed certain tests before we can definitely say that it has been recovered for the community; and we must therefore refrain at present from statistics, which would inevitably be incomplete and unreliable.

Here, now, is an instance of a *second son, ambitious, and inclined to steal* by a need for admiration (Lehndorff-Krauss).

Emile, twelve years old, is the second son in a family of five children (three older sisters and one twin brother). In infancy he had many illnesses. To-day he is tall and stout, precocious, and looks like an adolescent of fifteen or sixteen. When he was only ten, a neighbour took an outrageous liberty with him. He himself is very intelligent, and constantly quarrels with his brother whose mental development is decidedly backward. The two brothers sleep together. As he is very musical, Emile sings in the choir of a synagogue: for this he earns nine shillings a month, which he has to give to his father.

Troublesome symptom. He commits petty thefts, and he forged his father's signature upon a note sent by the schoolmaster about Emile's misbehaviour in school.

School report. In a general way his work is satisfactory, except in gymnastics and writing (a clumsy child).

Family. Bourgeois status, extremely ambitious. The father is very severe, and never satisfied with the children's progress, especially that of Emile in whom he has placed all his hopes. For Emile he sees a great future, one which will some day load the whole family with riches. The boy is very frightened of his father, and suffers much from never getting any praise from him. When he has some good report to announce, in no matter what subject, his father never fails to observe that he could have done still better. In this way the father has never recognized a single one of his son's successes; he chooses never to show what joy they give him; and this boundless ambition for young Emile acts as a systematic discouragement to him.

As for the mother, the transgressions of her child have put her beside herself. She is ready to do anything whatever if only it will lead to her son's reformation. The three older sisters work in an office, and the twin brother 'doesn't count' because of his weak-mindedness.

Profession. Emile would like to become a doctor, but his father prefers to see him as the great musician of the future!

Interpretation. Emile is an example of the type of child who is afraid of his parents and *deviates*, for lack of the courage necessary to rise above this feeling.

He believes that he is less well treated than his older sisters, neglected; and he grudges giving his father the little money he earns. He feels this state of things all the more since he was carefully pampered as a small child on account of his delicate health. And since his school successes have never won him the praises that he wanted to receive from his father, he is trying to play a part of importance outside the community. He conducts himself at school like a punchinello, and by that means manages to capture the attention of which he feels so much need. The *thefts* that he commits are a powerful means of keeping his mother on tenter-hooks about him, for ever since the day she discovered that he had taken something from her purse, she lives in apprehension that he will do the same to other people. In such bourgeois circles honesty is highly prized; it constitutes the supreme virtue, of which the least infraction is magnified into a crime. The child therefore naturally chooses this means of compelling his family's attention.

An over-severe upbringing has always this danger, since it may place the child between the two risks, of feeling crushed or of deviating from the path of communal life. The relationship between a harsh upbringing and subsequent delinquency is well expressed by Adler in the words: 'Druck erzeugt Gegendruck' (every compulsion engenders its resistance). In the majority of cases, a mania for stealing is, in a child, a sign of dissatisfaction with the affection and attention shown towards it. In every case one should inquire: from whom does the child steal, what does it steal and what does it do with the proceeds?

In the present instance, Emile steals money from his mother to give it to his comrades; a mode of behaviour frequently found in children who want at all costs to secure friends for themselves.

As for the forgery of the father's signature, it is a sure sign of the fear that this child feels towards its parents; for otherwise the act would be meaningless.

Treatment. First of all, we advise the parents to give their son a reasonable allowance of pocket-money, so that he shall no longer feel the 'need' to procure it in crooked ways. Purely external as it was, this was a measure that soon had a happy influence on the boy's relations with his parents.

Then we explain to them the relation between their over-severe pedagogic methods and the child's delinquency. We suggest that they should slacken the reins a little, to let him develop more freely, and we try to make them see the great danger of too ambitious an education. When a child feels that everyone in the family is expecting something extraordinary from him he is correspondingly discouraged by the smallest difficulty. His parents ought, however, to encourage him; they should not fail to praise him from time to time whenever he scores a little success. Only then will he be able to feel the beneficent and stimulating pleasure that comes from work well done.

Turning then to Emile, we point out to him that he can of course easily make himself conspicuous on the useless side of life, but if he wants to succeed in the future—whether he indeed becomes a doctor or takes to some other career— he will have to live within the community and serve it. For the present, what this means for him is that he should have confidence in his parents, who love him very much in spite of the mistakes he has made. They are so well disposed towards him that they are quite ready to grant him more liberty if they see that he is not abusing it, so why not show

them, from now on, that he deserves their trust? To stimu-
late his courage, we remind him that it takes more pluck to
ask his father to sign a disagreeable report than just to
copy his signature. Such appeals to courage, if they are
often repeated by the educator, gradually strengthen a
child's self-confidence and communal feeling, and help
it to give up the devious ways to which it had resorted
through weakness and lack of understanding.

Example of a spoiled boy who does not want to grow up (Löwy)

This is Henry, nine years old. He has only an elder sister
of thirteen, so that he is in much *the same situation as an only
child*, and is similarly spoiled. The sister occupies herself a
good deal about her little brother's education but, she says,
without success.

The father has been dead for some years. The mother, at
first most resistant to our advice, was completely converted
by what followed and was enabled to play an inestimable
part in her child's re-education.

Young Henry is brought to the council because of an
enuresia dating from his entry into school. He is wholly
dependent on his mother, and cannot dress himself or even
get up alone. From the medical point of view nothing is
wrong with him, but nevertheless the mother, after the
first visit to the council, insists on making him undergo
treatment at a clinic. She returns a few months later to tell
us that this treatment has had no effect.

We will transcribe the verbal exchanges in this case, for it
provides an instructive illustration of the transformation of
a mother. It also shows how it may be possible to treat a
child without speaking to it about its unpleasant symptom
(a procedure especially favoured by Fräulein Löwy). This has
the advantage of directing the child's attention elsewhere,
away from the bad habit on which it was concentrated.

Profession. Young Henry wants to be a teacher.

Favourite occupation. Building with a 'meccano'.

School reports. A timid child, rather passive, with a lack of interest in learning.

(*M.* = mother, *C.* = consultant, *H.* = Henry.)

M. (returning after three months' absence). He still wets the bed. I am in despair about it. I have to wake him every two hours at night to prevent it. It is unbearable!

C. The doctor having reported that Henry is in good health, we must look for a psychic cause of his bad habit. That is, we must try to grasp the unconscious end he is trying to gain by it. Probably your son has not much confidence in the future, his courage is low and he is trying with all his strength to hold on to the past, to the time when bed-wetting was allowable.

M. Besides, every morning he gives *me* (the pronoun locates the trouble!) endless bother about getting him up. He cannot dress himself alone and if I didn't always help he would never get to school.

C. I recommend an alarm clock, and that he be left to get up and dress by himself as a boy of nine should! We will speak to him about it. You can tell him that henceforth you won't help him; not that you're tired of it, but because it is necessary for everyone to learn how to dress himself.

We then suggest to the boy that he should not resort to his mother's aid except for things that he is absolutely unable to manage by himself.

C. Think about this, and tell us next time if there is anything in your behaviour that is now too childish. See if you find yourself doing anything that seems not quite suitable at your age.

(Next consultation)

M. Henry is taking swimming lessons. Perhaps that will

make him a little more courageous. I have to keep a sharp look-out, for he often tries to trick me. The other morning, when he had just looked at the clock himself, he asked me whether he would have to hurry to get to school.

C. You must bear in mind that what is expected of Henry is no less than a change of character. That is the hardest thing that can be asked of anyone; naturally, then, we shall need a lot of patience.

M. I sometimes think that Henry would rather not free himself from his faults, just so as to keep me constantly busied about him.

C. A very sound observation. Your son is beginning to gain independence, but he is still liable to slip back into his old attitude. These are his last tricks for attracting your attention.

M. That is not all. The other day when crossing the street he stopped in front of a motor-car, crying 'Look here, mummy!' I answered quietly that if he got himself run over I'd rather not look. I answered in the same way when we were out for a walk and he walked on the edge of a cliff asking me if I wasn't afraid he would fall.

C. You were quite right. Next time, don't say anything at all. He is now trying every means possible, to find one that will make you react as you used to. One has to allow children some time to assimilate any new idea. It is like giving an injection; you have to wait awhile for the desired effects. What one wants above all is to render the boy *independent*.

His sister complains of some bad turns he has done to his comrades. We explain to her that, despite appearances to the contrary, these are indications of progress, since the child was formerly too passive. If his newly-found activity is manifesting itself in a wrong way, the problem is to guide it in a socially valuable direction.

(Some time later)

M. He loves going to his swimming and I think he will succeed in it rather well. I would much like him to go regularly to a 'Hort' but he absolutely refuses.

C. (to *H.*). Wouldn't you like to visit a Play Centre just once, to see whether it would be nice just to go there, now and again?

H. No, I'm not going there. I don't want to.

C. Why do you think we ask all the children to go there?

H. I don't care why. I won't go myself, never!

C. You know, I think that those who refuse to go there even once are afraid. We all have to learn to live together. If you want to make friends you will be sure to find some at a Play Centre.

H. I'd rather stay at home with my playthings. If I went to a 'Hort' I wouldn't have any more time to play.

C. But you can take your toys with you. Many children do. Think about it until next time.

(At the following consultation)

M. When we got back, after the last time, Henry said 'I won't go to the Play Centre; I don't want to give up my free afternoons.' 'That's all right, let's say no more about it,' I answered him, but he persisted, 'If I don't go to the Centre you'll have some money left over, because there won't be the fees to pay. So you'll be able to give me more pocket-money—two shillings more . . .' I told him that was impossible; it had been hard enough for me to find the money for the Centre, though I would have made the sacrifice so that he might amuse himself with the other children. 'Well then, I shall take that money on the sly,' he said. I replied in the same tone 'But then I shan't have enough to pay for your food at the end of the month and you will go hungry.' 'I don't care if I do, because Margaret will have nothing to eat either,' he replied quickly, but then, after a few seconds of hesitation, 'Anyhow, I would like to go at least once to the circus.' I reminded him that we do go there once a year with Frau X and her children, but remarked that I would give him the money for it if he now wanted to go there alone. He made no answer. But he has been much better since that conversation, and for the first time for months hasn't misbehaved in the night.

C. Very good, you have already learnt a great deal. Say no more about the Play Centre. Later on, he may come back to that himself.

M. The other morning he complained of a headache and didn't want to go to school. I said to him 'Very well, stay at home.' At this he began to leap and shout for joy in his bed. I looked at him in astonishment and then quietly asked if he would not prefer to go to school at ten o'clock. And he did so, without a word.

C. Excellent! You ruined the good conscience with which he wanted to stay in bed! We must keep steadily in view the end we are trying to attain—to make Henry independent. The more so he becomes, the less he will need to fall back upon infantile symptoms and subterfuges.

(Some time later)

M. Everything is going much better, and any trouble at night is now rare. The other morning, when I did not praise him for having a dry bed, he asked me if I wasn't very glad to have so much less trouble with his linen. 'Were you doing it on purpose, then, all those other nights?' I asked him with great surprise.

C. Henry is now in full conflict with you. On no account lose confidence. Praise him now and again, just enough to help him to undergo the change more easily. The stronger he gets, the less he will need the help of others.

Several weeks then passed without any relapse. Henry's schoolmaster kept his sister informed of the boy's steady progress at school; he has become much more active, he works harder and better.

Here then, was a case in which a child was clinging most tenaciously to infantile symptoms, but whose transformation was made possible by the courageous attitude and patience of its mother.

Example of an only child, failing to establish contact with the community (Seidler-Novotny)

James. Fourteen years old; at college.

Father. A banker, finds no time to attend to his child.

Mother. Died a year ago. The boy's difficulties began from that moment.

James no longer works and frequently plays truant from college. He steals from his father not only money but even his watch, which he sold for money to go with some others to the cinema. He has a passion for the cinema and for sport: is interested in scarcely anything else. His school work going steadily from bad to worse, he will have to 'double' his class. Mathematics above all he finds too difficult. It is of interest, incidentally, that it is the spoiled children especially who do not succeed in mathematics. Dr. Adler attributes this peculiarity to their having done nothing by themselves, so that they do not know how to act, nor to think, independently, and it is mathematics, more than any other subject, which requires autonomous thinking.

James had been deeply attached to his mother, and in such a manner that he never undertook anything without her help. The disappearance of the mother when he was only thirteen was a terrible catastrophe for this lad, though in the end there was one good consequence; it set him on the road towards the community which hitherto had been completely closed to him. For no one now paid much attention to him from one day to another; no one now encircled him with warm affection, for the relation between him and his father had never been very close. The mother had not known how, at the right time, to detach the boy from her and to turn his interest towards the father and thence towards the community; that misunderstanding of her maternal function now made itself harshly felt.

This boy, who had never learnt to overcome his own difficulties, found himself stranded in a painful situation. At school he was soon one of the dull pupils and it had become almost impossible for him to change. At home there was no one to care intimately for him, his father being absent the whole day.

Advice. The father is advised to apply for a change of school for James. In a new atmosphere he will more easily pluck up courage to surmount the present difficulties. He will be in a situation where no one will know about his past, and if he makes but a little effort he will soon be among the better scholars. This is clearly a child needing to be relieved of a burdensome past.

The father being just about to marry again, we advise him at the same time to send his son to a boarding school for a little while, for a son whose attitude towards the father is already somewhat hostile would ill support the presence of a stepmother in the house. After a period spent outside the paternal home, during which his confidence and courage may be developed, the boy should be able to take his proper place in his new environment, the more so if we can profit by his absence and prepare the parents for his return.

We have noted already that Dr. Adler never willingly took a child from its home, his aim being to enable it whenever possible to adapt itself to given circumstances. But in exceptional instances (such as this where a new mother is about to replace the one who has disappeared) it may be preferable to send a child away until everyone concerned has been able to recover their equilibrium.

The consultant should then be able to judge the right moment for re-introducing the child to its family.

Example of a child suffering from excessive inferiority-feeling

The child. Bernard, seven years old, is in the first class of a primary school.

The mother. Very young, lives with her brothers and sisters.

The father. Nearly always occupied abroad, no one knows why.

Bernard is living all the while with adults. The complaint is that he is ill-mannered and truculent both at home and at school. His mother has to obey him like a slave, and he will not do his homework unless she remains seated beside him. The situation has become intolerable since little Bernard no longer wants to go to school, on the pretext that he already knows all that they teach there.

The psychologist therefore asks him, at the first consultation, if he will kindly help him by recording the proceedings. But Bernard replies that he knows only what they teach at school.

He is quite open to our explanations, which are intended to make him understand how many things he has still to learn which a child in the first class ought to know; how to be polite to his comrades, to listen to them without interrupting, to help his mother instead of giving her trouble.

Interpretation. We are in the presence of a child altogether unprepared for social life, incapable of living in a society of equals. He is suffering from a feeling of excessive inferiority, due to his having lived hitherto in a society of grown-ups, where he has, no doubt, often heard such phrases as: 'You are still far too young for' so and so. If he feels a need to behave badly toward others and disparage them, it is in order to lower them and to raise himself in his own esteem.

Advice. We offer the mother suggestions tending to the systematic development of her child's courage and independence. To this end Dr. Adler himself sometimes had recourse to a subterfuge: he would explain to the adults, in the child's presence and loudly enough for it to hear, that there are children who are unable to do their work unless their mother is sitting beside them. He added however that they are mistaken, not having realized that they have to become independent if they want to succeed in life, and that those who are at school ought already to be able to do their lessons by themselves and to behave properly to their schoolfellows.

Bernard listens and understands. His is one of those rare cases in which a palpable and lasting improvement can be observed from one day to another.

This *indirect approach* often succeeds very well in cases of intelligent but rebellious children; while direct admonitions may endanger the purpose of re-education by provoking yet another unfavourable reaction.

It is interesting to consider what a child entering the room for a consultation imagines it will be like.

Some of them have not the least idea what to expect, others think they have been brought because of a sore throat or a broken tooth. As a general rule, these children are the most accessible to the consultant.

It is more difficult to win the confidence of those who know that they have been brought to the council as a last resort. Their parents have often made them feel something shameful about this; creating an impression that all will be lost if the last means proves unsuccessful. There are parents who do not even scruple to tell the child that it will then end its days in prison.

In such cases the first duty of the consultant is to create, as quickly as possible, the initial confidence that is lacking. His task is even harder with these children, brought to him in spite of themselves, than with their parents who come of their own free will.

Example of a hated child (Wexberg-Seidler)

Marie. Thirteen years of age.

The mother. Blind and ill, has been bedridden for years. She can therefore do nothing for her children.

The father is an extremely brutal man. It is not by chance that he adopted the trade of a butcher. He adores his younger son: of Marie he takes no notice except to ill-treat her.

The eldest brother is eighteen. He has refused to follow the trade of his father who has turned him out of doors. Taking advantage of the parents' absence on a holiday, he broke forcibly into their room to burgle it. His parents themselves denounced him to the police.

The younger sister is pretty and a good pupil. She is spoilt by all the family.

Marie is on bad terms with her parents. She is afraid of them and suffers bitterly from being constantly reminded of the 'good example' of her little sister. It is a typical case of the hated child.

Her school work is below standard. She is so frightened of showing her parents her bad school reports that she goes so far as to falsify them. Nor is it surprising that she also commits petty thefts (of a comb, a handkerchief, etc.) from a schoolfellow.

One day, after having altered her report, she attempted to commit suicide by throwing herself into the Danube. Her schoolmistress, having heard of this some time afterwards, did not entrust the next report to the child, but asked the father to present himself with her at a medico-pedagogic council.

Marie is excessively discouraged because her little sister is at every moment preferred before her. When the two girls want to learn to play the piano, the father decides that the younger shall take lessons and then she can show her bigger sister what she has learnt! And so forth . . .

The attempt at suicide, the deceptions and petty thefts are so many means by which the child reacts to the lack of affection and the injustice of her parents.

Treatment. This child will not be reclaimed unless she can be reconciled to her parents and they can be persuaded to show equal consideration to both of the girls. It is moreover necessary to make Marie understand that it is for herself that she ought to be working at school, and not to please her parents. The success of her re-education will depend in the first place upon such contact as one can manage to bring about between Marie and her mother, for it is an ever-unsatisfied need for affection that has led her astray.

Example of a friendless child (Wexberg-Seidler)

Denise, nine years of age, lives with her aunt and uncle, on account of unsatisfactory conditions at her home (a very numerous family obliged to live in most inadequate lodgings). Her foster parents are very good to Denise, and it seems that she loves them too.

It is for her 'nervousness' that her aunt brings her to a council—a rather unusual reason in Vienna. In most cases the children are brought for some misconduct, for thefts etc.—in brief, for delinquencies that might embroil them with those about them, at school or in society. Most parents put off any appeal to the council until the last moment, for a remnant of false shame prompts them to dissimulate the misbehaviour of a child as long as they can. They need to be better informed on this subject, preferably by public lectures until they all realize that prevention is invariably easier than cure.

(*A.* = aunt,   *Dr.* = Doctor,   *D.* = Denise.)

A. Denise's nervousness takes the form of incessantly teasing and playing malicious tricks on her schoolfellows. She upsets the whole class by never keeping quiet for a minute; she quarrels with everybody and goes so far as to spit in other children's faces. At home she declines to do her duties so that I am sometimes obliged to punish her. She takes no interest except in gymnastics and dancing for which she is very gifted. And as you will see, she is a pretty child.

Dr. Have you any other children?

A. No, she is quite alone. We take great care of her and I am with her all day.

Dr. Has she any friends that she plays with?

A. No, she has no friends. I don't allow her out to play, because she has her household duties to do and they take her all the afternoon. (School hours are only from 8 to 1 in Vienna.)

Dr. But what does she do besides go to school? A good deal of her time must still be free.

A. She practises on her piano.

Dr. Don't you think she may want to see her parents, and brothers and sisters?

A. No; when I threaten that if she won't obey I will send her back home, she begins to cry.

(The aunt now withdraws and Denise enters the room)

Dr. What is your friend's name?

D. (after some hesitation). Alice.

Dr. Would you very much like it if she sometimes came to the house where you live, or if you went to hers, to play with her?

D. I'd like it very much, but auntie wouldn't let me.

Dr. Are the children nice to you?

D. Yes.

Dr. But you sometimes do silly things and then your schoolfellows don't like you. Will you try to be a little more gentle to them? If you settled down to work with the others, you would very quickly find you liked school. I can very well understand that you dislike it if you're not living in peace with the others. If I were in your place, I should do my duties quickly. Then you'd see that you would have plenty of time left to play with your friends. You are nine years old now. That means you are big enough to know how to divide your time. Would you like me to ask your aunt to allow you to invite a friend?

D. Yes.

Dr. Do you know already what you would like to be?

D. Yes, a dressmaker.

Dr. Then you'll need to be able to do arithmetic, to measure the stuffs and to draw. Think about all that some time in class.

(Denise having gone out, the aunt comes back again)

Dr. Denise is very biddable, she has quite understood what we have explained to her. From now on she will do her work expeditiously, and it would be good for her if you would allow her to go out afterwards to amuse herself with a friend. She needs contact with other children, which is the best education of all. Don't talk to her too often about her duties. What she needs is to learn to take responsibility for them herself, so that she may gain independence. And I shouldn't tell her she is pretty, she knows it too well already; rather point out that there is no merit in that whatever.

A month later this girl's school work is much better, but the aunt says she is less docile about the house. The aunt understands, however, that she must exercise patience and have confidence in Denise, who cannot alter herself all at once both in school and at home. The essential thing is that she makes progress, that her forces are not left inactive and that she is moving over to the side of the community. What matters most with a child is not its docility, but its activity and its productiveness.

Example of an over-severe upbringing (Wexberg-Seidler)

Ronald, aged twelve, has to stay another term in the same class 'because he is lazy'. Abnormalities excepted, we know that laziness is almost always the sign of an exceedingly discouraged child. It is brought on by some defeat, or by want of success and commendation. Idleness signifies loss of self-confidence, withdrawal from the struggle for lack of courage. It offers a convenient shelter, which does not bring discredit on the intelligence, for the child gives those around it to understand that 'I could if I would, but it is not worth my while to take so much pains for so little.'

'This child's difficulties are concerned only with mathematics.' We have already mentioned the relation that Adler finds between weakness in mathematics and want of independence. 'Ronald is the youngest of three children of whom the two older are already earning their living'.

Youngest children may show marked ambition and activity in some particular pursuit which removes them from any comparison with their elders; alternatively, they may intrench themselves behind their discouragement in a kind of passivity tinged with bitterness, with the idea that they can never equal their older brothers and sisters. The latter is Ronald's case.

'The mother is very severe with him. She means to replace the father—who has been dead three years—and employs the firm method.' We know what to expect from too severe an education, since every compulsion provokes its reaction.

In Ronald's case, the reaction consists partly in his idleness, and partly in the nervousness he betrays as soon as anyone speaks to him, even about subjects in which he is competent.

'Ronald is afraid of his mother, and this fear is the motive force behind all his actions.'

There is nothing astonishing in mediocrity of work done by a child who only works from fear of the cane. In that he will never find the incentive to overcome the smallest obstacle. 'He does not make the least effort when a difficulty presents itself. Even in music, for which he has decided talent (he plays both piano and violin) he shrinks from facing any obstacle.'

This boy has so strong a sense of inferiority that he continually mistrusts himself. His sole idea of work being that of something done under the constraint of fear, he naturally escapes from as much of it as possible. And the more so, the more corporal punishment is applied! This is a vicious circle, which must be broken before he will change his mistaken attitude. If punishments cannot be dispensed with at once, we must devise means to render them less often necessary.

Conversation between the Dr. and R. (a pale, timid lad)

Dr. Have you ever thought at all about the profession you wish to take up later on?

(No answer.)

Dr. Music?

R. I don't know.

Dr. How do you get on with your mother? Do you wish your relations with her were different?

(No answer.)

Dr. Are you afraid of her because she whips you?

R. Yes.

Dr. Do you find difficulties at school?

R. I can't do arithmetic.

Dr. Perhaps you don't take quite enough trouble because you believe beforehand that you can't do it. What do you do when the master calls your name?

R. I'm so frightened that I can't say a word.

Dr. And when one is frightened one can't calculate—that's quite understandable. But all this could be altered. If you like, you can be given some private lessons, under a teacher who will not set the tasks for you, nor will he punish you even if you don't work. He will simply help you and explain the things that are not yet clear to you. If you give yourself just a little trouble, you will then succeed very well. You want only a little patience and perseverance. Will you try?

The doctor afterwards explains to the mother that her son is so timid and discouraged that she had better not punish him at all, but on the contrary encourage him all she can, assuring him that he is as clever as the others, and able to do equally well provided he makes the necessary efforts. She should turn the lights up on any good result he attains and 'prepare' those little experiences of success that do so much to encourage a child. For it is only through 'visible' progress that self-confidence ever develops.

Interpretation. This child's timidity is such that it causes inhibitions extending even to the performance of music in which he excels. The problem is that of modifying his attitude to life. He is too delicate to stand the rough constraints of the education he has been undergoing; the fear which hitherto has been his motive force must be replaced by confidence and pleasure in work. Then the sanctions to which his mother has resorted hitherto will soon become needless.

Example of an upbringing alternating between excessive severit
and unhealthy indulgence (Adler's 'between the birch and the
sugar-stick') (Wexberg-Liebel)

Louise, thirteen years of age, is idle and stubborn. She
falsifies her school reports and believes herself to be in
capable of any success in studies. Very precocious, she i
carrying on an undesirable friendship with a girl friend
She was born in Czechoslovakia, where she passed her firs
two years of schooling.

The father is very often away and the girl has been brough
up exclusively by women.

The mother is inconsequential in her methods, which
oscillate between strokes of the cane and excessive indul
gences.

The difficulties began as soon as Louise came to Vienna
and they increased at the birth of her little brother.

This girl has vowed that she will become a dressmaker
She informs us that she hates men and that she would neve:
wish to have children.

Interpretation. We may regard her attitude towards the
opposite sex as a 'masculine protest' precisely in Adler':
sense. Viewed *externally* she is acting just as though she
meant to degrade the feminine rôle (she wants to be child
less) and were trying to do without men by being hersel
as like a man as possible. She is trying, by her relation:
with her friend, to convince herself that 'I have no interes
in men'. But viewed *from within*, this relationship is the
stratagem of a discouraged girl, haunted by fears of the
opposite sex; it is a measure of security against possible
defeats.

Her one-sided education has failed to equip her with the

necessary courage for life in society. And her failures at school derive from this discouragement, which no one noticed or helped her to compensate at the moment of her entering the German-speaking school. She had then to acquire another language in order to follow the lessons, a requirement that exceeded her adaptability. Her condition became worse with the arrival of the baby brother, for Louise envied the care and the affection bestowed upon him by the mother and felt she had been reduced to second rank. To attract fresh attention to herself she became obstinate and lazy.

By appropriate explanation, and by enabling her to gain experience in a real community, we endeavour to change her mistaken attitude and to reconcile her to her feminine rôle in life.

Example of a hated child deviating into complete immorality (Adler-Liebel)

Cf. *Int. Zeitschr. für I.*, p. 3, 1929 (Lazarsfeld).

As we have had occasion to remark, the *sexual problem* should not be treated apart, for it constitutes an integral part of the problem of education as a whole. An individual's behaviour in the sexual sphere cannot be isolated from his or her entire personality.

The *precocity* of a child is never sufficient, of itself, to explain sexual deviation, which is but rarely found except among children brought up without sufficient affection, and oftenest among the illegitimate, ill-treated and miserable. The family and social surroundings are of primary importance in these cases, and sexual deviation is the method that may be chosen by an adolescent who feels his personality is being stifled, to make himself feel better, to fulfil a need for superiority. For lack of courage, he cannot do himself justice and continue to live in accord with society, so he abandons himself to excesses that society condemns. (Let them hate, so long as they fear me!) Sexual misconduct is all the more effective, the more conscious he is of the capital importance attached to it by adults.

Maria. Fourteen years old.

Mother. Suffers from tuberculosis and a nervous illness.

Father. A drunkard and brutal.

Brothers and sisters. Three boys of twelve, nine and six years, and a little girl of two. Maria tyrannizes over all of them.

School. Her work is mediocre. Her compositions strike one by their unbridled and confused fantasy, sometimes by incoherent sentences. Very sensitive herself, Maria is a little flatterer, seeking to ingratiate herself with the mistress.

The latter greatly deplores the bad conditions at Maria's home and the brutality of her father. The girl is much too precocious and knows all about everything to do with sexuality. She was born out of wedlock when her mother was only seventeen. Whenever the mother has had to endure a night with the father she turns her bad temper against Maria. One day several pupils came to the teacher in great excitement about what Maria had just told them: that she had had intimate relations with a boy of thirteen as well as with one of her brothers; and that evening she meant to go out with some men. She had already several times spent the night in an hotel: she liked doing so and got money by it . . .

In the course of a subsequent talk between the mistress and the girl, the latter began by denying everything, but then admitted her enormities without seeming to see anything extraordinary about them. The mother, who was then called in, did not appear surprised beyond measure at what she was told. Her dismay was evidently feigned, and one had a definite impression that it was with her consent that

163

Maria was abandoning herself to prostitution. The mother added that her child was always lying and had already committed petty thefts.

When one tried to make the girl understand how wrong it was to have acted as she did, the attempt only increased her tendency to lower and denigrate everything in her surroundings. One could see that her behaviour both at home and out of doors, was inspired by one and the same *will to be revenged* upon those around her.

Her behaviour had reached the point at which Dr. Adler advised her expulsion from school, where she had become a danger to the other children. A reformatory school would hardly have improved her, since she would have been in the midst of other delinquents; Maria was therefore placed with a childless couple where she could be kept under constant supervision, and when she had become somewhat less a-social she began to frequent a Play Centre so that she should find herself in a community of children. We were unable to follow the development of this case any further.

Example of a child suffering from an organic inferiority (Adler-Liebel)

The danger of spoiling a child is considerably greater when it is ill. In illnesses of short duration a little exceptional pampering can hardly do harm, but with any chronic disability the problem is real. It may be difficult to put this point to a mother who is over-careful of her child because it has, perhaps, some real infirmity; it is nevertheless true that she would do better to bring it up as far as possible as though it were normal. It will suffer less from its physical inferiority if this is not constantly procuring it special treatment. The upbringing of such a child should tend to make it compensate—and perhaps over-compensate—for its organic inferiority. (Lord Byron, born with a lame leg, compensated it by swimming, and over-compensated it in the sphere of art.) (Cf. Chapter I, p. 7.)

This is the best way to prevent the child's becoming prone to presume upon its infirmity, as though this gave it the privilege of behaving a-socially, an assumption which maternal over-solicitude may easily reinforce. Really to help a child with an organic defect one must endeavour to bring it up as if nothing were wrong with it and make it follow as far as it can the normal course of education. By developing the faculties that are unimpaired with all its might, it will suffer less from the limitations imposed by its defect, and one can the better lead it to appreciate the possibilities that remain open to it.

We will cite here the case of a young girl:

Monica, thirteen years old, born out of wedlock by a mother of seventeen. The mother's parents turned her out of doors because of this, and she believed she was bound to marry her child's father though she already had no regard for him. Life with him soon became intolerable and they were divorced. Monica has lived since then alone with her mother, who is never tired of telling her that she loves her, adores her, that she is her only treasure in the world etc. Far from demanding anything of her, she waits upon her like a slave.

Monica's father was a syphilitic and she has been weak from birth. Already as a baby she suffered from a paralysis of the arms which however was cured: she now suffers from very weak sight and violent headaches.

Since her mother is constantly repeating that it is excusable for 'her poor child' to stay away from school, that she has a perfect 'right' to go there late in the mornings because she always sleeps badly at night, it is not surprising if the girl harbours feelings that are far from social and finds it hard to adapt herself to school life. The mistress knows about her state of health and treats her with indulgence, but the little girl presumes upon this situation and her conduct leaves much to be desired. She continually ridicules her schoolfellows and disturbs the lessons. Her work is poor and she has had to double nearly all her classes.

Interpretation. It is easily understood that Monica, in this situation, suffers much from the feeling of inferiority. This feeling has been fostered at once by her poor state of health, her family situation and the mediocrity of her performance at school. But her mother, instead of encouraging her to compensate for these unfavourable conditions, exerts a retarding influence upon her by inculcating the idea that the child has a right to privileged treatment. Hence the inability of this girl to make a proper contact with a society, her refusal to belong unreservedly to the community.

Treatment. Obviously the mother will have to rise above the feelings that attach her too exclusively to her daughter before she can try effectively to develop the girl's independence and assurance. And she will not be able to fulfil this condition unless the educator succeeds in making her understand the whole complex of relations that must be unravelled.

Example of a child that has lately undergone prolonged treatment in a hospital

(Cf. *Int. Zeitschr. für I.,* p. 3, 1931.)

Because of what they may have heard about hospitals, children sometimes enter them with feelings of fear or hostility. And since the nursing staff have often too little time, in the hospitals of great cities, to give very much attention to their little patients, a stay in hospital not uncommonly renders an a-social child more so than it was before.

Pauline. Eleven years of age, is the adopted child of a tiler.

Father. Dead.

Mother. Has gone away with another man, taking no more responsibility for her little girl.

Pauline has suffered since her second year with tuberculosis of the bones; she has been very ill for the last five years. She has spent whole years in hospitals and convalescent homes. At school (in a special class) and at home, they complain of her selfishness, her jealousy, her sensitiveness and her aggressiveness.

Interpretation. This is a child whose prolonged segregation in institutions for the sick has prevented it from establishing relations with the community. This has accentuated its feelings of inferiority and its envy of other children who enjoy more freedom in their movements.

Treatment. Pauline's school work being rather good, Dr. Adler advises her transfer to an ordinary class, with a view to giving her a little encouragement. Her foster-father is advised to have as much patience as he can with the little girl; to lose no opportunity of encouragement that may lessen her inferiority-feeling and inspire her with confidence. In this case it is the loss of her family in her earliest years which is at the bottom of the trouble, and life in hospitals has not supplied but accentuated this sense of deprivation.

Nevertheless, we know of many cases where the opposite has occurred; children who were unbearable at home have adapted themselves so well to the common life of the hospital that they have found within it, beyond all question, much of what is most valuable in a true community.

For instance, a little girl of eight writes from hospital to her mother: 'Don't worry at all about me. I've been here twenty-two days already but to me it seems like only ten.

I shall soon be able to get up, and then the time will pass quicker still. And then I shall be with you again.'

A child that gives such a description of its stay in hospital is evidently bearing its lot with patience, thanks perhaps to an understanding nurse or again to the little friends she has been able to find there. For cases of all kinds, the nurses need to learn something of psychology; and phrases such as: 'If you're not good I shall send for the doctor' need to be banished from their vocabulary. For any such appeal to higher authority betrays some lack of assurance in oneself. Similarly, the children should be made to feel, in every way possible, that each is the object of a sympathy felt equally towards all. Hospital life also offers to children innumerable opportunities to help one another, and how to turn them to advantage is one of the things nurses need to know.

We will cite another case (Friedmann) which illustrates *the important part played by the family situation* in a child's development and behaviour. This is a family which we had the good fortune to be able to observe intimately for the space of several months.

The mother and child presented themselves only once at a council. They did not wish to come again, perhaps because of the shocking scene which then took place between the mother and child or perhaps from fear of having to reveal things that are 'nobody else's business'. We know only that this family concluded that the council was an institution to beware of.

But as they were looking for someone to give lessons in mathematics to the little girl, we offered our services and were glad of a pretext that would enable us to enter into contact with this family and to improve, if we could, the situation of the children.

The father, an elderly accountant, had died in the previous

year from an attack of apoplexy. Invalided by the war, he had been unable to work during the last five years of his life and he had employed his leisure in the composition of little poems which earned him the admiration of the whole family.

The mother, still quite young, pretty and attractive, did not know to whom she should devote herself after losing the husband she had adored. Unsure of herself and inconsequent in her methods, she was on very bad terms with her children. She assumed that she must always be 'in the right', on pain of forfeiting her 'dignity as a mother' which she wished to safeguard at any price.

L., her daughter of twelve, is in the class appropriate to her age. Formerly a very good pupil, her school work has been poor for nearly a year, and is particularly bad in arithmetic. She remains good at drawing, gymnastics and dancing of which she is passionately fond. In the other subjects she is very lazy and follows the lessons without interest. Very jealous of her little brother, who she thinks is preferred before her, she makes use of him in all kinds of ways. The boy lends himself to her caprices, for he adores his big sister, but she herself will do nothing for anybody. Her distrust of her equals goes to such lengths that she thinks they are all nothing but liars, spies and flatterers, regarding herself as the exception that proves the rule! Not of a very cheerful disposition, she seems to enjoy nothing, unless it be a visit to the cinema.

Future profession. L. hesitates between that of a *kindergarten teacher* in which she could show her mother how children ought to be brought up, and that of an *author*, who would be able to teach her, by a book, how to treat children with equality and justice!

Her brother H. is very timid and afraid of adults; he suffers from having too little affection shown him. Unlike his sister, he very much likes housework, and already shows remarkable cleverness at it. As is often said to him—'It is you who are the girl and L. the boy!'

On weekdays he makes a fuss about getting up, whereas he is always the first to rise on Sundays. He hates school, is among the worst of the second-year pupils, and the master is continually threatening to put him back to first-year grade. Out of school, on the other hand, he exhibits striking abilities. He can recite by heart long pieces of poetry after hearing his sister declaim them but a few times. He sings well and amuses himself by writing little poems which he afterwards sets to melodies, also of his own composition; and all this although no one at home takes special notice of it.

The grandmother shares the home of the family. She is always suffering and her presence is a burden upon everyone.

The flat is small but neat. Each person has a separate bed, which is taken to indicate a certain measure of comfort in homes of this neighbourhood. What is pitiable in this family is an atmosphere of bitterness and constant mistrust that poisons the relations between its members. To take one example amongst many: One Sunday (we have mentioned the alacrity with which he rises on that day) H. goes quietly into the kitchen to prepare breakfast. His mother and sister are still asleep, and he means to serve them in bed, knowing that this pleases them. He decides to whip the top of the milk as he once saw his mother do, but, either because it had been skimmed already or was not quite fresh, the milk would not beat into cream . . . He was still struggling with it when his mother and sister, having awakened, called curtly for their coffee. The dejected H. brought it to them 'without cream'; and L., after moistening her lips at the cup, handed it back with a wry face, saying, 'Go on, drink it yourself. It's quite cold and nasty.'

The little fellow, who had risen early with joyful thoughts of the little surprise he was about to prepare (at only seven years old he could manage the gas stove by himself!) went back without a word into the kitchen, and there his mother found him an hour later, seated on a stool and still in tears. And even then nobody offered the least word of consolation to this little soul in distress.

The few occasions when we were able to get a talk with L. alone (for the whole family were usually together in the only room that was warmed) were enough to convince us that the girl was in that period of obstinacy which Charlotte Bühler calls the 'negative phase'. In full physical development, but before puberty, the child was in revolt against everything. (Cf. L.'s declaration about the kinds of professional career she imagined for herself.)

A few weeks later L.'s condition became still worse following upon a change of class at school. She had passed from a Class B to a Class A, a promotion which ought rather to have encouraged her. But she grumbled at her new surroundings, in which she thought some of the children were rich. This meant that she felt jealous of the few girls who were more expensively dressed . . . She showed a lack of energy and interest, and made no effort to follow the course of instruction or adapt herself to her new situation. She preferred to assume the pose of the idler who flatters herself with the illusory idea that 'I could if I would but it's not worth the trouble'; when in reality she does not dare to try for fear of a failure.

During the lessons in mathematics that we were giving her, we were struck by this girl's quickness of understanding. And when we asked her why she did not do the same work equally well at school, she replied:

'I've heard it said that there are some people who send out "rays", and that they make everyone around them able to do whatever they ask of them. I think you must be one of those people!'

But to her surprise we at once endeavoured to lead her to admit of a less mystical and more understandable explanation. We explained to her that she had too strong a desire to have other people giving her their exclusive attention, that she was refusing to be only one pupil among the others and was trying all the time to play a part by herself. We proceeded to show her that it was because she did not achieve brilliance in her school work that she was trying to content herself by playing the part of an idler, one who needed to be specially persuaded to do what the whole class had to do as a matter of course; otherwise she would strike some attitude to amuse everybody and make herself the centre of attention.

L. had a sense of the practical so well-developed that she wanted to learn only what was sure to be useful to her in later life. She often asked us whether a good knowledge of arithmetic was really necessary in order to become the mistress of a kindergarten.

Interpretation. L. is a discouraged girl, barricading herself behind a wall of laziness. She would like always to occupy some extraordinary position, and acts as if she could succeed in doing so without making the least effort on the communal side of life. The striving after superiority, by which she is unconsciously making up for her feeling of inferiority, naturally shows itself in her attitude to anyone who is weaker—her little brother. Although he has never had a word of thanks from her, he dares not refuse her anything; whenever his big sister commands he feels bound to obey.

Treatment. First of all, it is necessary that L.'s forces should be set in motion, if we are to transform her passivity into productive activity. She will have to admit to herself that it is impossible for her to achieve anything whatever without personal effort, and that the feeble consolation that 'she could if she wanted to' will never satisfy her. But it is not by words that one will ever convince her; only by appeal to her own living experience.

We take recourse to little exercises, designed to direct her too-egocentric attention towards other persons. For instance, we advise her to take notice of those around her and try to see the good side of each of her schoolfellows. After a little of this, she asks herself for the first time what would give them pleasure; she discovers that she can be of use to them and thus makes herself friends. At last she has the joy of finding herself reintegrated in a community the existence of which she had never before realized.

This transformation was made possible only by the aid of the whole family. As soon as the mother wanted to give her help, the family atmosphere became much better and mutual confidence began to revive.

As for little H., he was in great need of personal strengthening and encouragement. The reason for all the trouble he gave about getting up in the morning was simply that he detested going to school: he showed no such reluctance on Sundays. His bad school record was almost wholly due to his discouragement, his master being unable for want of understanding to give the boy what he could not find at home. One little event illustrated particularly clearly the effect of fear upon a child's school work.

The master was always complaining of H.'s handwriting, which looked like the scribbling of a five-year-old. So, when the little fellow was about to do his homework, we asked him to write the first line of the page as well as he possibly could, but said that he could do the rest just as he liked. (This is a trick invented by Fräulein Löwy.) At the end of half an hour, the child showed us, with great pride, a page neatly written from beginning to end! We asked him why he had not limited his carefulness to the first line only, and he replied, 'Because that wouldn't have looked pretty with the rest. So I thought it would be better to do the whole page properly.'

We saw then that this boy wanted only a little praise and recognition, and he would soon take his place among the good pupils.

We mentioned the part played by the mother in the general improvement that we were happy to record. After a certain length of time she made herself more indulgent to everyone. She ceased comparing her own children, continually and always to their disadvantage, with those of her sister, and refrained from telling them that it would have been better had H. been a girl and L. a boy. Better still, she got to the point of making them understand that it was just as good to be either a boy or a girl, and that it is only our own actions that can do us credit or the reverse.

We applied ourselves methodically, in the case just cited, to carry conviction more by deeds than by words. For it is beyond question that to live through an experience teaches one more than the cleverest explanation of it. And if we finally managed, as we hope we did, to render these children capable of self-education, the abortive initial consultation did not, after all, fail of its purpose.

In the chapter that was devoted to the experimental school, we saw that its work could not be limited to the education of the children; that in the nature of things it had to be extended to the re-education of parents. Since such re-education is clearly impossible without individual treatment which the school itself cannot undertake, it devolves inevitably upon the councils. Without denying that there are other educative methods which may banish troublesome symptoms, we remain convinced that the radical reformation to which we and many others aspire is attainable only through a treatment that is highly individualized, and for this a deeper knowledge of the child's family is indispensable. To become a genuine centre of such education, the school therefore needs to avail itself of advisory councils, and to act in the closest collaboration with them.

CHAPTER FIVE

Critical Observations

No one who has been able to estimate, at first hand, many of the successes achieved by the use of Dr. Adler's ideas will ever minimize the importance of the work of this great psychologist and philanthropist. Whoever has once heard him speaking to a father or mother in distress, or to a child that had lost all confidence, will have been permanently convinced of the profound truth that was living in him. Of his deep feeling also, his love for mankind. It was this spirit, united with a very sure knowledge of men, that gave him such swift insight into the suffering of those who came to him for help or advice. Nobody every knocked at his door in vain. With an equal sympathy toward all, he was an unfailing friend of the people.

His great activity, based upon strong convictions and a profound desire to better the condition of man, was the secret of his success. For living example will always convince men more effectually than the most eloquent discourses about the necessity of mutual aid or the feeling for community.

We are living in days of great moral and economic disarray, when men are often overwhelmed by doubt and the conditions of life have become tragically precarious. Confidence is shaken and men are aware that they are passing through a fundamental crisis. Neuroses, psychoses and crime—an epoch that knows too much of all these varieties of deviation cannot but welcome a discipline whose essential purpose is to give human beings a new confidence in their destiny, renewed faith in their mutual responsibilities. All of those—alas, so many—who have strayed from the way of community are discouraged souls, wounded and distrustful, led into wrong paths through some defect in their earliest preparation for life. In such paths they continue to go, to train themselves or even force themselves, until at last despair or an utter weariness brings them to standstill. Their suffering itself may then be an occasion for good, for in no other way would a radical change become possible. But for the goad of despair, few if any would ever humble themselves to seek the aid of the doctor or psychologist.

A. UPON THE THEORY

Adler's psychology applies to all, since it is always, in the last analysis, from the same evil that human beings suffer—from lack of faith in themselves and in others. This genial and—as his detractors so often say—oversimplified view of the matter is the basis of Adler's inestimable work as a re-educator. Admittedly, one is at first tempted to object that this method is only a generalized scheme, despite its claim to be a psychology of individuality. But one is not long in finding out that the methodology is only a frame of reference within which one is able to relate all the difficulties and deviations possible, and estimate them as symptoms of individual failures to fulfil the threefold task of life (duty to others, duty towards the opposite sex and the demands of one's occupation). The apparent formalism is merely instrumental; it in no way detracts from the individuality of each case under consideration but, on the contrary, places it in a setting of sufficient scope.

The greatest and most reassuring thing about this method is that it does not stop at the elucidation of the errors in an individual's style of life; it goes on to make him understand

N   177

them. By perseverance in re-education and resourcefulness in counsel, it guides the subject into the way of life that is right and natural for him, showing him how he can do better than he has done hitherto.

We have all experienced the truth of the poet's words—*Video meliora proboque, deteriora sequor* . . . It is not enough to point out the right way, one must help those who have strayed from it to regain it. And if they are to be rendered capable of following, without some fresh deviation, the path they have last recognized as right for them, their first steps have to be guided and upheld. This path, as we have seen, is the one that leads them to the community through the strengthening of their own personality.

We have also seen how Adlerian psychology always seeks to take full account of existing human relations. Thus understood, psychology relates itself closely to sociology and indeed becomes inseparable from it. Man is not only an individual being, nor only a social being but both at the same time. We all suffer from the contemporary discord between individual and society, which is not only an individual matter; in our days it is convulsing the whole world. It is Nietzsche against Marx, or Nietzsche against Fascism . . . Adler's psychology, the central problem of which is that of the individual's relation to society, is thus especially representative of the preoccupations of our age, and at the same time it constitutes a generous attempt to transcend the crisis of our culture. It is for future generations to pronounce judgement on its value.

It is always interesting to look for the currents of philosophic thought by which the author of a psychology has been consciously or unconsciously influenced. In this respect *Adler's* name has often been linked with *Nietzsche's*. At first glance the points of resemblance are indeed sufficiently striking. One may say, in the first place, that if the

philosophy of Nietzsche both continued that of Schopenhauer and reacted against it, Adler's psychology occupies
much the same position in relation to Freud's psychoanalysis. Similarly, the transition from Freud to Adler, like
that from Schopenhauer to Nietzsche, is a movement from
pessimism to optimism.

Adler and Nietzsche, no less than Jean-Jacques Rousseau,
believed in the original goodness of man, of whom they had
the highest hopes. Both the one and the other responded
to life with a courageous 'yes' followed by 'in spite of
everything' ('trotzdem').

But in noticing these resemblances we must not lose
sight of the divergences. They both tell us much about the
'will to power' (Machtstreben, Wille zur Macht); but this
will plays very different parts in their respective conceptions
of the world. For Nietzsche, as we know, it constitutes the
very essence of the living being, the condition of its 'self-
surpassing'; whilst for Adler the will to power is only a
psychological reality which has to be reckoned with in
order to canalize and direct it to the community. And from
this point the divergence widens: Nietzsche, the aristocrat,
preaches a 'master-morality'. Addressing himself only to
an élite, he glorifies the *amor fati* of the individual as pure
self-reliance and self-attainment, and he celebrates the
generosity and 'bestowing virtue' of the individual ego.

Adler, the democrat, desires on the contrary to improve
the conditions of the mass of men: for him the affirmation
of life has value only in so far as it is harmonized with the
exigencies of a community moving ever more and more to
the ideal. If the personality of an individual achieved its
highest possibility of development, it would still remain
incomplete so long as it maintained itself apart from its
responsibilities to the community.

For Nietzsche, freedom is a necessary illusion, an

invention of the ruling classes for the use of the crowd. Man is neither free nor responsible for his actions. Nietzsche does not believe that man can ever know himself, for his instincts are impenetrable and he is condemned to perpetual ignorance of the springs of his actions. For the philosopher of the 'will to power' the idea of community is devoid of all meaning, altruism and compassion are only feelings of weakness. In these opinions Nietzsche is as completely opposed to the fundamental virtues recognized by Adlerian psychology as to those of Christianity. Appearances notwithstanding, the philosophy of Nietzsche remains, in our view, essentially negative, because it denies the existence of spirit and of freedom and affirms the fortuitous. But it is through his spirit that man participates in the infinite. This was well understood by Adler, whose psychology embodies the fertile notion of final causality. This is, indeed, the originality of his method, and as it is the point upon which it is most often attacked, we think it worth returning to. But first we must say a few words about the part played by *fictions* in the psychic life.

Adler often speaks of the 'fictive goals' (fiktive Zeile) that the individual so often sets himself, thereby blinding himself to what he really ought to be doing. As this term easily gives rise to misunderstandings, it is important to perceive its exact meaning.

A misguided child, no less than a neurotic, may set itself a fictive goal. A child may want to play the part of its father and identify itself with him: a neurotic may be trying to surpass and excel 'everybody' by his deeds, knowledge or ideas etc. In the one case as in the other, we are of course confronted with a fallacious attitude to life from which the individual has to be set free before he can be brought into positive contact with the community. But what about the man who is well-balanced? Adler admits that he too may have recourse to fictions, but with this vital difference—that in his case the fiction serves him only as the means to a goal that is concrete. He entertains his fiction so long as it is required by the end in view, but without being enslaved by it. In a healthy man, his fictions are indeed a kind of working hypotheses, which he is prepared to abandon when they no longer correspond to any reality. They enable him to orientate himself in the world, but they never develop into ends in themselves.

It is a great merit in Adler to have demonstrated that the life-style of the neurotic is illusory because it revolves around the fictive goal, which is a self-delusion. And here again he resolutely turns his back upon Nietzsche. Nietzsche believes, in effect, that illusion is necessary and ought to be fostered in the lives 'of the masses', while Adler desires, on the contrary, to see them delivered from it. As we have just said, he allows fictions as means in the normal man, who always knows how to entertain reservations about their ultimate value. And we are inclined to believe, for our own part, that here too the path of progress is from the fiction to the truth, from a fiction gradually reshaped according to a truth more and more fully realized. It is not a case of finding the way most convenient to follow, but rather that which leads most nearly to the truth. Who knows, moreover, whether the two will not one day coincide?

Adler is frequently reproached for having introduced the principle of finality into his psychology, as the motive force of individual development. But this conception follows naturally from the way that he envisages a man as a unity to be grasped only in its totality. It is in this that the Adlerian system marks an advance upon the causal conception that is characteristic of psychoanalysis. By this conception, too, Adler enables us to bridge the gulf between a naturalistic view of the world and its spiritual significance. Viewed in the light of causality, there is nothing in the world that was not pre-determined from its beginning and we cannot logically be held responsible for a single one of our actions. The individual no longer can be said to perform them, he is much more like 'the field of battle on which the instincts contend for supremacy' as Künkel once remarked about psychoanalysis. This leaves no room for freedom, for responsibility or for creativity, and it is no exaggeration to say that determinism excludes life itself. Its kingdom is one of necessity under efficient causes into which man cannot enter without previous mutilation. That is why Adler appeals to the notion of finality, for to him, man is genuinely the author of his own actions and always responsible for them. When one asks of an individual why he behaved precisely in this or that manner, there can be no satisfactory answer if it is related only to the past. For the real motive is always a goal that the man proposes to attain. When an infant cries we are told that from the causal point of view, he is crying because he is hungry. From a finalist standpoint, on the contrary, we say that he is crying in order to procure nourishment. That trivial instance admirably illustrates the difference between the two conceptions, the one mechanical and the other vitalist. In the former case, the relation between cause and effect is one of necessity. The same cause, under the same conditions, will always produce the same effect. In the second, on the contrary, the relation between the means and the end is one of freedom: the same end might be attained by the most diverse means, just as the same means might be used to achieve very different ends. A child may cry to inspire pity. It does not at all follow that its crying will always mean the same thing, and whenever it cries one has to look for the end to which its tears may be the means.

Every end, as soon as it is achieved, becomes in turn a means to the attainment of a further and higher aim: and so on to infinity. This is what Künkel calls the '*in*finale Betrachtung'. For him, the deeper significance of 'finality' is the infinite.

Another criticism of Adlerian psychology is that it seeks to discredit the *factor of heredity* and empties the words *talent, gift and aptitude* of all meaning, by affirming that all individuals possess the same possibilities at the moment of their birth. It is true that a few Adlerian psychologists have not scrupled to proclaim this opinion, but our business here is with their original teacher, namely Dr. Adler himself.

He confirmed, as a physician, the truth that is now generally admitted (without remembering who stated it for the first time) that very frequently it is not the illness that is inherited but the disposition to it, the organic inferiority, the environment. Adler never intended to deny that heredity may impose limitations upon the development of an individual; what he rightly contradicts is that these limits must of necessity make the individual a-social. In theory he confesses to ignorance about the mysterious thing called 'talent'; but only to draw our attention to the fact that, in practice, this is a question in no way deserving of the importance so commonly attached to it. Beside the primordial influences of example, imitation and nurture, he regards heredity as a secondary consideration. Hence his fundamental optimism, his confidence as an educator and his unshakeable faith in the destiny of humanity. But, it is asked, what of genius? Adler admits freely enough that training alone is not enough to explain genius. But geniuses are exceptional, few of them born in a century, and the problem therefore hardly concerns him. Is not his attitude confirmed, moreover, by the words of Goethe, 'Ist Genie nicht nur Fleiss?' (Is not genius only application?)

To pass to a very different objection—if one considers all the different attitudes which, according to Adler, an individual may assume towards the duties that life imposes upon him, one may at first be struck by the absence of examples of those that are 'sane' and 'normal'. Their absence is however natural, considering the point of departure of this psychology and is no argument against it. Born of psychotherapy, Adlerian psychology was necessarily concerned with the scientific investigation of all the attitudes that it found to be characteristic of individuals whose sense of community is defective, a deficiency not compatible with the healthy attitude. For the healthy attitude is that of confidence, of the courage with which an individual tackles the three great tasks that life presents to everyone. This last objection, by the way, could usually be raised concerning any educative method of a therapeutic origin (Montessori, Decroly).

B. UPON THE PRACTICE

The actual work of Adler and his disciples extends far beyond its theoretical foundations, as yet little developed. As we have had several occasions to remark, it is the practical side of this psychology which chiefly interests the educationist.

We can make only brief reference to the kindergartens that are working upon Adlerian principles. The few that so far exist in Vienna are only at their beginnings, and there is room in them for much further improvement. Besides the replacement or continuation of familial education and the preparation of the children for life at school, kindergartens present the immense advantage of bridging the gulf between social classes. We may even regard them, in this respect, as a factor making for peace; for the experience of friendship, of living together in frankness and mutual helpfulness in this very early stage of social life, constitutes an initiation for these little ones from which much may be expected.

But the institution which comes nearest to realizing Dr. Adler's ideal is certainly the experimental school. We have seen what marvellous results it obtains, in the teeth of deplorable social and economic conditions, thanks to the ability and the conviction of its staff. There are two points upon which we find fault, though we are far from blaming the school management, which has no power to remedy them. These are the division of each class into sections A and B, the objections to which outweigh the advantages, and the exclusion of any subject touching upon sexual questions. The removal of this *veto* would break down an important barrier between pupils and teachers.

After having intimately followed the remarkable work accomplished in this school, we felt but one thing more we should desire; and that was to see the example of the three pioneer directors imitated by all the other masters on the staff, so that the school might still more fully constitute a single consistent experiment and convince an ever-growing number of educationists.

As for the Adlerian psycho-pedagogic councils, one can hardly formulate criticism, even of a summary character, of institutions that differ so much both in procedure and results. Whilst all of them originated in the ideas of Adler, some of them diverged, and not always with happy consequences. This verdict must be supplemented by another which may seem sufficiently commonplace; namely, that the success of a method depends largely upon the person who is applying it—or thinks he is. It must be admitted that some of the Adlerian consultants furnished ammunition to Dr. Adler's adversaries and even gave rise to criticism by his friends. But these embarrassments should not be allowed to detract from the work of those who know how to put the ideas of Adler into practice with excellent results and whose researches contribute to the continual improvement of the consultative method.

On the whole, the results obtained by the councils are good. They would be better still if the councils in the different neighbourhoods collaborated more closely, for each would then benefit by the experience of the others. Their financial resources being almost non-existent, all the work has to be done without payment and the psychologists can make no exacting demands upon those who lend them benevolent assistance. It is none the less necessary that these collaborators should be selected with greater care, in the interest of the treatments undertaken. These are weak points upon which the councils cannot be commended. They are not grave, but they ought to be remedied as quickly as possible, for they supply arguments precious to Dr. Adler's detractors; the more so because men are all too easily inclined to judge of a whole movement by the least of its members. A man who has been robbed by a Chinese is all too ready to say that the Chinese are thieves!

One feature of the consultations that is often under attack, not always unjustifiably, is their partial publicity. In its favour Dr. Adler urges that a council ought to be a place where all those who are devoted to education can learn; for them it should provide a school of practice in the management of difficult children. It is at these councils that beginners should be enabled to take their first steps in that immeasurable domain of knowledge—the knowledge of human nature. Moreover the councils should increase their understanding of the misfortunes and sufferings of those who come to them for advice and deepen their sympathy with all, without distinction of class.

For the child, too, the public consultation is not without

advantages; the interest taken by a number of persons in what is preoccupying the child relieves its feelings of isolation. It sees other children there who are suffering from some difficulty like its own, and the symptom for which it has been brought to the council is no longer felt as something exceptional. It must be added, too, that the consultations are only public up to the age of puberty, to about the age of fourteen. After that, the young adolescent speaks with the consultant alone.

But the publicity also holds dangers for a child. Its vanity is often flattered by expressions of interest in its troubles, and then it may want to play up to its audience by 'putting on an act', tragic or comic as the case may be. On the other hand, a child may easily be distracted by the presence of the other persons; then it sometimes wants to know what they have come for; and this may give the consultant much more trouble in establishing the necessary contact.

Lastly, many impressionable children are intimidated by an array of persons unknown to them. They are shy of speaking; it is sometimes impossible to get a word out of them; or they exaggerate or distort the facts without meaning to do so.

It is true that the consultant can obviate these dangers in some measure by monopolizing the child's attention as much as possible in order to establish the required intimacy. Many of the psychologists make the child sit facing them with its back turned to the auditors. This is often enough to make it forget their presence. It is also a common practice for the parents to whisper in the ear of the psychologist whatever they want to tell him.

But more important than anything else is that the child should carry away from the consultation the impression that it has been understood, that it should go home with a feeling of relief. To ensure that result a psychologist needs outstanding qualities; above all plenty of tact, an ability to sound, with the most delicate discretion, the childish soul that has come to confide in him; and he must know how to refrain from all curiosity and misplaced criticism.

We conclude then, that the public character of these councils does involve certain dangers which ought not to be ignored, and that much depends upon the consultant's knowing how to obviate these dangers if a consultation is to yield all the benefits foreseen by Dr. Adler.

C. COMPARISON WITH OTHER METHODS OF CONSULTATION

Before leaving this subject we wish briefly to compare the Adlerian councils with other consultative methods that we have been able to study closely.

Of the different *psychoanalytic* clinics at Vienna that of Dr. Aichhorn is the most noteworthy. We were privileged to attend it regularly although it is usual to admit only those who have been psychoanalysed and are desirous of practising psychoanalysis. We should add, incidentally, that in Vienna one need not necessarily be a doctor to be able to practise psychoanalysis.

Generally speaking, the cases presented at this clinic are examined from the three following points of view:

(1) Is this a child that should be taken out of its present situation and placed in the care of the child-protection service?

(2) Is this a child that should be subjected to a daily analysis?

(3) Is this a child that should be re-educable at the clinic itself (which is held once a week)?

Cases of the first kind rarely come back to the clinic. They are handed over to the bureau for child-protection.

Those of the second category amount to between 20 and 30 per cent of the children and young people dealt with at the clinic. Dr. Aichhorn confides such a patient to the care of the one of his assistants whom he regards as the most competent for that particular case, telling him to undertake an analysis and report progress every week.

But it is in the conduct of those cases whose re-education Dr. Aichhorn undertakes at the clinic itself that one is able fully to feel the intuitive powers of this extraordinary man, this sagacious judge at the tribunal of childhood who so often seems to grasp the whole tragedy of a human situation at a single glance. No less than Dr. Adler, he lays special emphasis upon the indispensability of educating the parents. But whilst Adler seeks first of all to induce the parents to modify their attitude towards their children, Dr. Aichhorn invites them to visit him together and tries to bring them to a better mutual understanding. However, this comes to the same thing in the end, for in the one case as in the other it is the harmony required for the development of the child that one is trying to bring about. Aichhorn, like Adler, draws the parents into conversation, listening most attentively and without interruption until they have said all they have to say. Now and then he resorts to the method of free association, or he may ask them for memories of events that they have lived or dreamt.

As for theory, his conception of man is determinist. He asks in any given case: 'What caused the a-social attitude of this child?' But in an entirely natural way he supplements this conception by what is in practice a finalist considera-tion, for he always takes account of the objective which a child is seeking to attain.

As we have noted before, psychoanalytic consultations are never public. They take place however in the presence of some others, generally of four to six analysts desirous of instructive material. From time to time Dr. Aichhorn lets them know by a sign that he wishes to remain alone with the child or its parents; they then immediately efface themselves until after the latter have departed, when Dr. Aichhorn acquaints them with what he has learnt in their absence.

In practice then, and with the exception of the cases it is decided to submit to analysis, this psychoanalytic method of dealing with parents and children differs much less than the theoretical divergences of the two schools would lead one to expect. The psychoanalysts too are trying to liberate the individual from a burden of the past, in order that he may courageously face the difficulties before him. But here, and once again, everything depends upon the personality devoting itself to the psychoanalytic work.

As for the medico-pedagogic clinic of the *Institut des Sciences et de l'Education* at Geneva, opened in 1913 and directed to-day (in 1935) by Dr. Brantmay and Mme. M. Loosli, it is committed neither to Adlerian psychology nor to psychoanalysis, but follows a kind of 'free method'. This begins first of all with a medical examination, and such information from the school and the family as the assistants have been able to procure. Then it proceeds to the educational problem as primarily an individual one. It willingly makes use of the Terman test in judging the development of a child's intelligence, and of the Rorschach test for judging its affective life. Upon the basis of these investigations the child is then guided in the manner most conducive to its own development.

With regard to the parents, these workers limit themselves to the giving of a little advice, never venturing to propose a complete change of attitude after the manner of the Viennese consultants. In this connexion it must however be noted that there are as yet no regular reunions of parents at Geneva; it is therefore more difficult to interest them in educational questions. On the other hand Geneva is in advance of Vienna in having a well-managed home for the observation of cases, which forms an invaluable complement to the clinic.

D. CONCLUDING OBSERVATIONS

For Adlerian psychology really to become, as it intends, a complete design for living it would have of necessity to be founded upon a *transcendent principle*. It is true that the idea of community, as Adler conceives it, is a transcendent ideal to which man continually aspires without ever being able completely to realize it. But Künkel sees more deeply into the problem when he tries to establish a relation between Adler's psychology and Christianity, between the idea of the community and the duty of loving one's neighbour. That would open up a vast field of debate, beyond the scope of this modest treatise, about the relations between psychology and metaphysics. Meanwhile, the practical task, the task of the educationist, is how to make a child understand that one sees, over and above itself, a higher principle; that of the spirit in its infinity.

Since example speaks a language more convincing than the most eloquent praise, we will add but few words by way of conclusion.

Dr. Adler had a genius for the practical; he was a man of action to whom the highest duty of life was to come to the aid of all those who suffer, to unravel their errors and to rekindle the light of confidence within them: a man through whose efforts thousands of individuals lost in devious ways have been restored to the community. Not from his personal ambition, nor from any desire to form a school, have his teachings inspired so many disciples throughout the world.

It was his vigorous optimism as a re-educator that enabled him to succeed with the most difficult and inveterate cases: his indestructible faith in the fundamental goodness of man that made him able to bring about personal reformations which an age more mystical than ours would have revered as miraculous.

But far from taking the merit to himself, Alfred Adler remained a modest man, well aware of the endlessness of his task, and with reverence before the mysteries revealed to him in every day of his busy life . . .

Bibliography

ADLERIAN PSYCHOLOGY

ADLER, ALFRED, *Understanding Human Nature*. Trans. by Walter Béran Wolfe (Geo. Allen & Unwin, London, 1929).
Practice and Theory of Individual Psychology. Trans. by P. Radin (Kegan Paul & Co., London, 1924).
Problems of Neurosis. A book of case histories. Edited by Philip Mairet (Kegan Paul & Co., London, 1929).
The Neurotic Constitution. Trans. by Bernard Glueck (Kegan Paul & Co., London, 1921).
The Education of Children. Trans. by Eleanore and Friedrich Jensen (Geo. Allen & Unwin, London, 1930).
The Pattern of Life. Case Histories of American Children. Ed. by W. Béran Wolfe (Kegan Paul & Co., London, 1931).
Studie über Minderwertigkeit von Organen (Bergmann, Munich, 1927).
The Case of Miss R. The Interpretation of a Life-story. Trans. by Eleanore and Friedrich Jensen (Geo. Allen & Unwin, London, 1929).
The Case of Mrs. A. The Diagnosis of a Life-style (Individual Psychology Publications, Medical Series, C. W. Daniel & Co., London, 1931).
ADLER, ALFRED und JAHN, ERNST, *Religion und Individualpsychologie* (Passer, Vienna-Leipzig, 1933).
ADLER, FURTMULLER, WEXBERG, *Heilen und Bilden* (Bergmann, Munich, 1928).

BIBLIOGRAPHY

ADLER, ALEXANDRA, *Guiding Human Misfits*. A Practical Application of Individual Psychology (Faber & Faber Ltd., London, 1939).

BIRNBAUM, FERDINAND, *Die Seelischen Gefahren des Kindes* (Hirzel, Leipzig, 1931).

DEUTSCH, LEONHARD, *Individualpsychologie im Musikinterricht* (Steingräber, Leipzig, 1931).

DREIKURZ, RUDOLF, *Seelische Impotenz* (Hirzel, Leipzig, 1931.)

HOLUB, ARTHUR, *Die Lehre von der Organminderwertigkeit* (Hirzel, Leipzig, 1931).

LAZARSFELD, SOPHIE, *Technik der Erziehung* (Hirzel, Leipzig, 1928).

RUHLE, ALICE and OTTO, *Schwer erziehbare Kinder, Schriftenfolge*. Edit. Am andern Ufer (Dresde-Leipzig).

SCHULE und LEBEN, *Individualpsychologie und Pädagogik* (Mittler, Berlin, 1927).

WEXBERG, ERWIN, *Individual Psychological Treatment*. Trans. by Arnold Eiloart (C. W. Daniel & Co., London, 1929).
Sorgenkinder (Hirzel, Leipzig, 1931).
Individual Psychology and Sex. Trans. by W. Béran Wolfe (Jonathan Cape, London, 1931).

BY VARIOUS AUTHORS, *The Contribution of Alfred Adler* to psychological medicine, the study of organic inferiorities, questions of the relations of the sexes, general medicine, etc. (Individual Psychology Publications, Medical Series No. 19, C. W. Daniel & Co., London, 1938).
Internationale Zeitschrift für Individualpsychologie (First 11 years 1923–33 published by Hirzel, Leipzig. Twelfth year 1934 published by M. Perles, Vienna. Reappearing at Vienna since 1947).

PSYCHOANALYSIS

AICHHORN, AUGUST, *Verwahrloste Jugend.* Intern. Psycho-analytischer (Verlag, Vienna, 1925).

FREUD, SIGMUND, *Introductory Lectures on Psychoanalysis.* Authorized Trans. by Joan Riviere (Geo. Allen & Unwin, London, 1949).

FREUD, ANNA, *The Psychoanalytic Treatment of Children* (Imago Publishing Co., London, 1946).

OTHER WORKS RECOMMENDED

ANDERSON, H., *Les Cliniques psychologiques pour l'Enfance aux Etats-Unis et l'oeuvre du Dr. Healy* (Delachaux et Niestlé S.A., Neuchâtel, 1929).

BAUDOUIN, CHARLES, *Suggestion and Autosuggestion.* Trans. by E. and C. Paul. (Geo. Allen & Unwin, London, 1920).

BLEULER, *Lehrbuch der Psychiatrie* (Springer, Berlin, 1918).

BOVET, PIERRE, *The Fighting Instinct.* Trans. by J. Y. T. Grieg (Geo. Allen & Unwin, London, 1923). *The Child's Religion.* Trans. by G. H. Green (Geo. Allen & Unwin, London, 1940).

BUHLER, CHARLOTTE, *Das Seelenleben des Jugendlichen* (Jena, 1925).

CLAPARÈDE, EDUARD, *Experimental Pedagogy and the Psychology of the Child.* Trans. by Mary Louch and Henry Holman (Edward Arnold, London, 1911).

DESCOEUDRES, ALICE, *Le Developpement de l'Enfant de deux à sept ans* (Delachaux et Niestlé S.A., Neuchâtel). *L'Education des Enfants anormaux* (Delachaux et Niestlé S.A., Neuchâtel).

DOTTRENS, ROBERT, *L'Education nouvelle en Autriche* (Delachaux et Niestlé S.A., Neuchâtel).

HETZER, HILDEGARD, *Kindheit und Armut* (Hirzel, Leipzig, 1929).

KÜNKEL, FRITZ, *Charakter, Liebe und Ehe* (Hirzel, Leipzig, 1932).

Eine Angstneurose und Ihre Behandlung (Hirzel, Leipzig, 1932).

KÜNKEL, FRITZ and DICKERSON, ROY ERNEST, *How Character Develops* (C. Scribner's Sons, New York, 1940).

LOOSLI-USTERI, Marg., *Les Enfants Difficiles et leur Milieu familiale* (Delachaux et Niestlé S.A., Neuchâtel, 1934).

NIETZSCHE, FRIEDRICH, *Complete Works* (J. N. Foulis & Co., Edinburgh and London, 1909–13).

SPRANGER, EDUARD, *Lebensformen. Geisteswissenschaftliche Psychologie und Ethik der Personlichkeit* . . . Vierte . . . Auflage (Halle, Saale, 1924).

STERN, L. WILLIAM, *Psychology of Early Childhood up to the sixth year of age*. Trans. by Anna Barwell (Geo. Allen & Unwin, London, 1924).

General Psychology from the Personalistic Standpoint. Trans. by Howard Davis Spoerl (Macmillan & Co., New York, 1938).

Index

A

Abnormal child, distinguished from the normal by absence of plan of life, 21, 106; treatment when socially intolerable, 104–06

Active school, the, 52, 60, 63

Activity, importance of, in progress of child, 158; ruled by idea of community, 60

Adler, Dr. Alfred, philanthropist and psychologist, 176; comparison with Nietzsche, 178–82; his point of departure from Freud, 1; educational success due to his optimism, 4, 192; optimism based on belief in educability, 11; experience at a collective conversation, 107; ideal most nearly realized in the experimental school, 185
See also Adlerian experimental school; Adlerian psychology; Medico-Pedagogic Council

Adlerian experimental school, comparison with State schools, 75–6; equipment needed, 77–8; examinations, 56; ideals are autodidacticism and co-operation, 78; method incorporates other methods, 77; self-government, 63–4; reports, 57–8; success achieved in spite of adverse material conditions, 49–50; re-education of parents, 174

Adlerian psychology, essential aim, 59; basis for pedagogy, 37; central problem of, 178; criticisms of, 177, 181, 183; one of finality, 4, 5, 36; heredity, 9–11, 183; one of individuality, 177; man conceived as a totality, 2; preventive func-

tion, 34–6; related to sociology, 178; therapeutic function, 33–4

Adler-Liebel, report of the hated child deviating into complete immorality, 162–4; report of child suffering from organic inferiority, 164–6

Administrative community, 63–4

Admiration, need for, leading to theft, 141

Affection, lack of, causing sexual deviation, 162–4

Aichhorn, Dr., psychoanalytic clinic at Vienna, 188–90

Anderson, Dr. H. H., Account of the Healy psychology clinic, xi

Apperception, 'tendencious', 23

A-sociality, defective reasoning the distinguishing characteristic (Birnbaum), 106

Attitude, importance in cases of inferiority feeling, 8; its importance in Adlerian psychology, 41; a. of the mother determines the baby's behaviour, 125; objective attitude imperative for psychologist, 115, 120–1; 'Autistic thinking', 40; Autodidacticism, 78; Autonomy, best instrument of education, 84

B

Baudouin, 'Diana complex', 24; 'castration complex', 25

Beethoven, instance of compensation, 8

Behaviour, relation between bad work and bad behaviour, 136

Binet, scale for measurement of intellectual capacity, xii

Printed and bound by CPI Group (UK) Ltd, Croydon, CR0 4YY

01/11/2024

01782630-0002